CU00869259

A Brain Tumour's Travel Tale

Visit my website at https://auntymbraintumours.co.uk/

Dedication

To my Mum for being there as my rock, Camilla and
Reka for putting up with me.

Acknowledgements

I thank God, who has brought me through the good the bad and the ugly. I wanted to give up on him and on myself on many occasions, however he told us 'Cast all your anxieties on him because he cares for you.'

Thank you to my friends and family for your patience and your love.

Thank you so much to Doctor Minhas and his surgical team at St George's Hospital.

Thank you to the Croydon Community Neuro-rehabilitation Team, Doctor von Oertzen, my seizure specialist and Attend ABI (Acquired Brain Injury) support team.

Thank you to everyone on Aunty M Brain Tumours for allowing me to do something I am very passionate about.

Content

Introduction

I'm not going to lie to you, I am no Jane Austen. Nevertheless, I'm hoping you will enjoy finding out a bit about me and finding out about my brain tumour. An Intraventricular Meningioma (that is a tongue twister if I ever heard one).

First things first, here is a quick ride down memory lane so you know where I came from and who a few people in my book are.

I was born on Wednesday 27th March 1983 at around 12:00 noon. I was two months premature and only 4lbs 5oz. Aahhh! Tiny – right? Anyone who knows me would know I certainly made up for my shortcomings as I am 5'11" now. The rushing into everything didn't really change much in my life. Well, until Wednesday 21st May 2008 when I was diagnosed with a brain tumour.

I wanted to introduce a few people first as you will see them in the book. Starting with my parents and my brother. Mum and Dad met in a bikers' club and are both huge bike enthusiasts. They were married in 1973, and both had good careers. My mum was in Media and Events, and my dad was a Money Broker up in the city. They had my brother in 1981 and moved to what is now our family home in London in 1983. Ian my big brother (aka 'Smelly'; he calls me the same thing, so it is not as bad as it sounds and also, we really don't smell, well I hope not anyway). Ian moved to Sydney in 2007.

We have lived next door to the same families all the time I was growing up. Our neighbours on the right side had two children, Emma and Blake, who were nearly the same age as Ian and me. Emma is more like a big sister as she is a couple of years older than me.

I went to boarding school when I was eight years old in 1990, and this is where I met my best friend, Camilla. In 2002 I met my other now best friend, Reka. You will see these girls a lot in the book.

You will hear about Roland who I met when I was in College and also Becca and Naomi who I met while in college.

You will meet Clare and Amanda and a few other ladies who I worked with at Petro-Canada, an oil and gas exploration corporation.

Finally, I will tell you about my company Aunty M Brain Tumours which I set up in May 2011. I will tell you all about that soon.

OK, so! Those are some of the people you will see in my book. I have always had journals since I was 6 and I tried to keep up with them even when I was unwell. So, I am going to share my journey through my diary entries with you. I won't write everything as there is 10yrs worth, it will get boring for you, so I have just pulled out the relevant bits.

The journey to where I am today wasn't easy. It was horrible. Many times, I sat down and wondered just what the point was, what kind of life did I have?

For me, finding something to focus on and to set as a goal as well as helping other people in the same position as me, has been such a positive thing to do and has given me a reason to keep going, no matter what

Just to set the scene... I did some travelling in Australia in 2006, and when I came back in April, I got a job with Origin HR an in-house recruitment company. I was put into the Dresdner Kleinwort account, I was enjoying my life, and there were no complaints.

The Story of a Headache

It was June 2006, and I had just come back from being in Australia for three months. I was looking for work in London and was approached by Origin HR, an HR outsourcing and resource management service. I was brought in to work on the Dresdner Kleinwort account, in the recruitment team. The first year was great, and I was thrilled to be there. I had a wonderful boyfriend called Will and was very content with my life,

In 2007, I was going on holiday to see my brother in Sydney in August for two weeks. and then one morning in April 2007, I was on the train during the rush hour going to work. One minute I was strap-hanging with the best of them, and the next I had fainted. Two men helped me off the train and onto the platform. One of the men said, "You may have an iron problem." I thought "Yeah, that must be it." The other man said, "You might be PREGNANT!!" I laughed and said, "No."

All of the passengers and the train driver were peering out the windows at me and wondering what was going on, impatient to get on with the day. I was wondering what was happening too. Embarrassed doesn't even begin to cover it, mortified is how I felt. I just remember willing the train and all those gawping faces to move off!

I called my mum and asked if she could pick me up and go to the doctor with me. While I waited for her, I called work to explain what had happened and say that I would be late. I told the doctor what happened, and they said it must be an iron problem and gave me some ferrous sulphate tablets.

Then, one weekend in August 2007, I was driving down to see Will in Reading and to meet his dad for the first time. His parents live and work in Dubai, and his dad was over in the UK for a visit. I drove down the motorway in heavy traffic, eventually arriving in the countryside. A colossal festival/concert was going on near his house. It took me around four hours to get there instead of the hour I'd expected, but I was quite happy sitting in the traffic, listening to music. It was a bit of an experience and very entertaining watching people, some of whom had given up waiting in their cars and had started to walk to the concert – all in high spirits, some quite literally!

My eyes went blurry while I was sitting in the car, and I thought that I just needed to stand up for a bit. I noticed that my hands were shaking and put it down to being hungry. Eventually, I made it to my boyfriends house. I felt terrible about taking so long to get there. I was trying to seem relaxed as Will did all the introductions with his dad. We went to a pub, but I couldn't hear anything people were saying. At times like this, you really want to make a good impression on the parents and not look too crazy. I kept smiling and hoped for the best!

After that weekend, I took a two-week holiday to visit Ian in Sydney. I was so looking forward to seeing him. By this time, I still had the shakes and was quite bad tempered, but I was not getting headaches. Ian and I had a great time over four days at the Gold Coast, Surfer's Paradise. It was the first time we had spent that much time together since we were children and it should have been good just to hang out. I could feel myself getting stressed about ridiculous things, but I tried to make the most of the break and didn't tell anyone how I was feeling. I just didn't feel right.

When we returned to Sydney, it was a public holiday and Ian, and I packed our bags and jumped into the car for a camping trip in the bush. It was fun. My eyes would occasionally go fuzzy, but I thought it was probably just my contact lenses not coping with the hot weather. After 14 days, I said goodbye to Ian and came back to London.

In September 2007, I was sitting in the office. We were all going out for a big dinner and to an awards ceremony. I said to my supervisor that I wasn't feeling too good and that my vision was a bit strange. I thought I should go home. She said it was essential that I be there and that I would be fine (I think I could have done with assertiveness lessons at this point). I just couldn't see it properly. It was just like having tunnel vision, my head in a box. All I could see was through a small area of tunnel vision to the front, with no peripheral vision. I asked God for help to get me through the night. I found that if I sat still my vision would start to come back.

My boss wanted to chat. She asked, was I happy at work? I said yes, but my headaches were getting worse. I was always having to snack when I felt faint and taking migraine tablets frequently. My boss said I should go back to the doctor, as there was apparently a problem.

I went to the doctor first thing the next morning who suggested I might be stressed and advised me to take a week off work. I hated it. I really don't like letting people down. I explained to my boss, and I was feeling awful about the whole situation. I stayed at Will's house for five days, as it was quiet there during the week. I spent a lot of time watching TV and random movies. I was so bored and aware that I must seem to be a bit crazy, but I couldn't explain anything. I was beginning to get depressed. I felt I had let my work down. I was so angry at myself and so unhappy. I just wanted to be alone.

Just before Halloween, Will and I decided to go to a Fright Night in Thorpe Park. We got there quite early, considering the park would be open until late. We went on one ride, and I was left literally shaking. I didn't know why, because I loved rides. I didn't want to look bad as it was my idea to go there, so we went on another, and I could feel that my body did not want to be there at all.

My migraine came on, and I thought it was just from stress and the loud music in the park. Knowing the park would be open for some time, we went back to the car and had a short sleep, hoping that I would feel better afterwards. That seemed to help, so we went back into the park and decided to go into the haunted house. All we had to do was walk through the house and past actors who jumped out at us. Easy. I am such a scaredy cat usually, but this night all I was focused on was a headache and the pain and thinking "If you touch me, I might just bite back." This time, the long one-hour queues were great for me because I knew I was not looking forward to more rides. It was quite scary not to have any control over my nerves. I really couldn't understand what was wrong with me.

I went to work the next day, and I was still moody, emotional and stressed all the time. In November I spoke to my boss and said I thought I was not right for the job as I was unhappy with all my problems. I left at the end of the month. I had already booked a holiday with Will to Dubai to visit his parents. I thought that it would be an excellent opportunity to get away from work and have a new start when I came back. I went to the doctor first, and he agreed that it was probably stress and that the holiday would be a great idea, but that I should relax and shouldn't overdo it.

It was so frustrating because, at the GP surgery, I never saw the same doctor. I always saw a different one. It felt like I was just a number and they were not really listening to what I was saying.

In Dubai, I loved the sun. The late mornings helped as well, as my headaches seemed to happen mostly early in the morning. I found it hard to relax though and spent time just lying in the sun always wondering what was going on in my head.

One day we woke up early to go with Will's mother to visit her company. His mum is the head of nursing in Dubai at the Canadian Hospital. While we were waiting to meet her, we went outside, and I was not feeling right at all. As we were walking back into the hospital, I felt very sick and faint. I was trying so hard to relax although, I knew what was about to happen – AGAIN!! The next thing I knew, I was on the floor with Will trying to pick me up with one hand and holding all our bags in the other.

It was just like the first time I had fainted on the train. Both times I had a quick dream – nice ones doing something like shopping, and then I opened my eyes and then I was just embarrassed. I was so thankful I was at the hospital already and, with Will's mother being the head of nursing, I was well looked after. They took lots of blood tests. I honestly think God was making sure I was in the right place, but nobody thought to give me an MRI. I told them I had terrible migraines. I was asked the usual, could I be pregnant or was I anemic. I was becoming so unhappy and fed up with feeling like it was my fault and all in my head or not look after myself and allowing myself to become anemic. I knew I was skinny then but not from dieting. I was so not enjoying myself and was thoroughly fed up, and I'm sure Will was as well at this point. I just wanted to crawl under a rock and hide and sleep, then wake up back in my home.

I had spent some of the holiday emailing employment agencies regarding new opportunities and I set up three interviews, ready for when I came back. From the three meetings, I was really interested in two of the companies. After three interviews with Brown-Forman and two with Petro-Canada, I was very excited when they both offered me jobs. I decided Petro-Canada was a better choice. I started on December 17th, 2007 and was so happy with my decision. I was providing administrative and secretarial support to a floor of thirty people including five MDs.

Petro-Canada was a crown corporation of Canada in the field of oil and natural gas. It was headquartered in the Petro-Canada Centre in Calgary, Alberta. I was working in the London office at London Bridge. I had the most fantastic view over the River Thames. I felt really blessed for the opportunities I was getting.

The job was going great, but in my personal life, I realised my memories and my recollections of everything were starting to disappear, and I was feeling very helpless and depressed. I couldn't separate my thoughts and was always angry inside. It was terrifying. I was scared.

At the beginning of December, I went to Will's friend's wedding. The wedding was as lovely and romantic as a wedding should be. After the ceremony, I said I needed to go to bed as my head was thumping as always. I couldn't move. I stayed in bed all night and then couldn't wait until the morning and go home. I could see Will was irritated by me and I felt I had let him down for not making more of an effort with his friends. I dropped him off and then drove back home to London. I was starting to feel spaced out again and was getting beyond fed up with myself and everyone else.

I went to a family friend's wedding on 30th December and took Will with me, and again I needed to sleep all the time because I was always tired and getting migraines. The relationship with Will was not working anymore. I was tired of feeling guilty for getting ill.

Around Christmas, I was at my worst. I started waking up in the middle of the night and having the most agonising headaches. I had never felt anything like it. It was like somebody was grabbing my head and slamming it against a concrete wall. I tried the usual tablets, but nothing touched the pain. I could only cry and pray that it would stop soon.

I was in so much pain, I would be sick. Night and day were just as bad as each other. I would dread waking up and just hoped that if I could get up early enough, the pain would go before I went to work. I have to say, with everything that was going on with my body I wanted to stay away from everyone. It was clear over Christmas that Will and I were not getting on well. We broke up at the beginning of January.

All my efforts were poured into my new job. I really liked the people I worked with, and I would always try to go for a quick drink after work, never staying too late as I knew it could easily lead to a headache, and I didn't want anything to go wrong.

I managed to handle all the strange things my body was doing and tried to adapt.

One night I went out with two friends to a roller disco. I was really looking forward to it, but when I got on the roller skates, I had never been so unsteady. I was really, off balance like I would fall down at any time. My stomach was spinning. I had to hold on to something. My body was quivering. It was so weird. I had to come up with an excuse to leave as I didn't want to explain how I felt.

My shaking hands got worse during March, and, as the doctors couldn't find anything wrong other than my migraines, they thought it must be stress again. I decided to go on holiday for 11 days with Emma to Dubai because we knew it would be scorching and we had friends out there. We also thought it would be a great break as both our relationships had recently broken up and it was coming up to a bank holiday and my 25th birthday. We had a great time, but Emma and I soon realised I was becoming very aggressive. It was never a problem, but it was noticed by both of us. I was getting slightly worried about my behaviour. I felt like I was boiling up quickly and not coping with noise or conversations.

One evening we went out and met some friends. We had planned to spend the day with them, but I'd needed to sleep as I felt drained and very weak. I thought I would be OK for that evening and said that we would find them later in the town. When I woke up, things felt a lot better. I made sure that I always had water with me and assumed that the heat made me weak. We had another great evening and Emma, and I had a great holiday despite me saying some strange things. Back home in the UK, my aggressive behaviour escalated. I was getting angry so quickly. I found it more straightforward just to stay away from most people so that I didn't offend anyone.

At the end of April, my parents went to Australia to see my brother in Sydney and my uncle in Adelaide for five weeks. I said goodbye in the morning and then went to work. I didn't really want to tell them of all the strange things that were going on as I didn't want them to worry when they were on holiday.

I was just looking to God for help. I spoke to my Pastor's wife and explained what had been going on. Sister Gill was concerned, and we prayed over the situation. I thought I was having a breakdown because even though I had no idea what that feels like, I thought it must be similar. I just couldn't explain what was happening. My memory was getting worse, and I couldn't even remember if I had eaten meals. I was finding it hard to hold a conversation because I would forget what we were talking about. It looked like I was just tired, but I knew it was something else.

That Saturday, I went out dancing with Becca. I was really spaced out again. My vision was strange, although it did eventually go back to normal. We danced the evening away, and then went home. The next morning, I didn't go to Church because I felt I had a bad attitude. I was fed up with my headaches every day. Becca and I had planned to drive to Brighton, but I could feel a headache coming on. I gave Becca my car keys and said she should drive. I had travelled that road for years and directed her to what I thought was the easiest route from home.

An hour later, we were lost. We did eventually make it to Brighton and had lunch on the beach. I couldn't believe I had got the directions so wrong. Luckily, we made it home. I had planned to have an early night, but I was just seething with frustration.

I called Camilla to tell her how I was feeling, and my hands were shaking, and when I was trying to speak, I didn't sound English. I was just gibbering on. By the end of the call, I managed to pull myself together. But things were becoming scary. I didn't know who I was.

When I was at work, I would use my hands a lot to express myself, which I have always done and used now to try to cover up words that wouldn't come out right. One day it was terrible. I remember working on a Friday and wanting to go home, but I was determined to make it through the day. All of my bosses were going to a big meeting abroad and would be away from the whole of the next week. I was talking with a colleague and having a giggle, but I was in a lot of pain from a migraine. I still can't believe I made it through the day and was able to get all my work done.

I had arranged for my friend Reka to come over for dinner but realised that I could barely move, let alone cook. Reka was waiting at the door for our girly night in. Reka was happy to cook dinner, and I had already put the food in the fridge in the morning. I lay on the sofa and just waited for the pain to go away. Then I was feeling a bit better, and we watched a film called 'PS I Love You'. This was a random selection, and it was the first sad and depressing film I had seen in months. I had been avoiding them after I broke up with Will.

The film is about a young lady, Holly, and her husband, Gerry, who were a happily married couple until he succumbed to a brain tumour. Even though Holly was broken-hearted, she was helped through it all by her friends. It really made me think about brain tumours and hospitals and friendships. I loved it, though I really didn't know why because it was depressing. I watched it three times with different friends. I found the film really calming – somehow, I think I knew something was going to happen but that I didn't need to worry about it.

On Monday 19th May 2008, I woke up at the usual time and, knowing that there were no managers around at work that day, I was able to make sure I had everything sorted on my desk. I told my colleague Abu that I was going to the doctor on a Tuesday morning. I was determined to get to the bottom of the headaches, the shaking hands, moods, my vision – just everything. I said I should be back to work in the afternoon. I was praying about everything every second of the day.

The following day I woke up early, waiting for the doctor's surgery to open at 08:30. I called my parents and Ian, as it was Ian's 27th birthday. I thought it was pointless to worry them yet; they were thousands and thousands of miles away. I said I was going to the doctor but didn't go into details. I just said that I had a migraine, wished Ian a Happy Birthday and put the phone down. I managed to get an appointment for 09:30.

I drove down to the clinic and went in for my appointment. I could feel that I was rude and demanding, but I was not in the mood to be shrugged off like every other time.

The doctor looked at the list of symptoms I gave her, and she said, "I don't know what is wrong with your vision, but let's get your periods sorted first and have your contraceptive implant taken out of your arm as that may explain your moods changing." The implant had been inserted in October 2007 to try and regulate my periods, but it wasn't doing me any good. I said this was not enough because I had the headaches before my implant (the implant has rods that release a steady dose of one hormone only – progestogen). The doctor insisted I should have the implant removed first and we could sort the other things after. I didn't want to wait and decided to go to Croydon to get my eyes checked by my usual optician.

There was time to spare, so I took my car to get a wing mirror that had been hit the week before sorted out. On the way there my vision went funny – it kept blacking out and then coming back all in the space of a millisecond. I had noticed that had happened once or twice when I was at work a few days before but thought it was because of the weekly sunbed I had had to top up my tan from Dubai. I blamed myself and decided that I would never go on a sunbed again. I was calm even though I had no idea what was going on, and I just prayed I didn't hit anything.

My vision came back, and I called my friend, Roland, who had turned up in England the day before from Hungary and was at home for two weeks. I think that when you are still and alone, you suddenly realise that God has already given you all the tools that you need for life. Just open your eyes. I felt capable of handling anything and had everything I needed. Roland was only two shops away from me for his own eye check-up. We met for a quick coffee, as our appointments were both in 30 minutes. I told Roland what had happened, and he said to call him after my appointment to let him know how it went.

The optician and a lady took some X-rays of my eyes and checked them. The optician asked for a second opinion. I could see she looked concerned. She said that she thought that it might be cysts in both eyes as there was bleeding in the back of them. She asked me to go straight to St George's Hospital and said that she was going to call them to expect me. I called Roland, and I told him what was going on, and he came straight over and took me to St George's. Although he could see that my situation was not looking good, he spent most of the time trying to make me laugh. I phoned my work colleague Abubaker again and explained what was happening and asked him to let my boss know if he asked about me.

We were waiting for ages. Roland was telling me all about his wife who was heavily pregnant and how excited he was about birth. After sitting for hours in the hospital, we met a lady who had a look at my eyes. She put some dye in them. She said it may be a cyst and she would book me in to see herself and her boss the next morning first thing in Mayday Hospital. She said I might be putting pressure on my spine and the fluid would need to be removed. At this point, I had dark yellow dye in my eyes, and couldn't see anything. I guess I thought it was my eyes that were the problem and thought I might lose my sight. It was frightening.

We drove back to my house, and I was drained from the whole day. I texted my parents to let them know that I may need to have an operation but didn't go into too much detail as I didn't really have any answers and didn't want to panic them. Roland said he would come back again later, so I gave him a house key. I cooked a basic dinner and then spoke to Camilla and told her what had happened. I lay in bed and prayed all night. I felt lonely until I prayed. I felt like it was a film and I felt sorry for whoever was playing me. Still praying I finally fell asleep.

'I'm very, very sorry.'

On Wednesday 21st May, I woke up and Roland was already downstairs. I phoned my colleague again to update him in case my bosses asked about me. Roland and I took some food with us as we knew how long these things could take. We were praying about everything. We spent the whole day in waiting rooms laughing, even though we suspected that we were not going to hear good news. God's strength kept me very positive for the whole day, and if I shut my eyes, Jesus was there smiling and saying, "Don't worry." I saw three different doctors, including the lady from the night before. They were prodding and looking at my eyes. They still thought I had a cyst and they wanted me to have an MRI scan later that day.

First, I had to go to one other doctor to run some more tests. At that point I wasn't really with it. Roland just took care of everything. I do remember the doctor had a bit of an odour problem, no offence, but he was very, very smelly, and he looked like one of those old doctors who may love their job but doesn't particularly like people. We had to try hard not to gag. The doctor was looking at my eyes and said he would get an MRI scan set up and some blood tests too. At that stage, I thought that I might have to wait for an hour, go home and come back the next day to look over what I needed to do. Roland lived close to the Mayday Hospital, and he went home to get some stuff done as I was going to be waiting for a long time. It also meant that he could park my car at his house instead of paying for the hospital car park fees. I sat there for two hours, during which time, I texted Camilla and Becca. It was feeling very surreal like this was happening to someone else, and I wasn't sure what this cyst would mean. I just kept praying and kept positive.

Eventually, I had the MRI scan. It was very daunting as the camera was an inch away from my face. I shut my eyes – it was so loud. Tears were streaming down my cheeks and for the first time that day I was scared, really scared. I suddenly heard a voice saying, "I'm here." I couldn't move, but I knew God was there. He smiled at me and said: "Not very nice in here is it?" He stayed with me the whole time. I felt so protected. I knew I needed to remember that he was there all the time. The crazy thing was, that day I was not in any pain, it was just all very confusing, but I knew I wasn't going through it alone.

I left the scan room and went to have some blood tests. I was just calling Becca and Camilla to update them when a lady ran over and said: "Hi, is it Claire Bullimore?" I said "Yes." She took me back to the part of the hospital I had been to before the scans, and I waited to be called in. An old lady was waiting as well as an old man and a couple. The older lady was offering everyone sweets, and it was making me laugh talking about her piles, but I soon lost my appetite.

An hour later it was just me and the couple waiting. I had a feeling couple were Christians; we talked about our Churches and about God. The wife went to a Pentecostal church. Her husband went to a Church of England church. He was saying he didn't like all the singing and jumping around at a Pentecostal church. I said I love singing and dancing, so it was perfect for me. Then they went into the doctor. So, after waiting two hours I was the last person. I genuinely believe God let me meet some great characters in the waiting room to stop me sitting there and worrying.

The doctor finally called me. I was relieved that they must have found something rather than sending me off with nothing. The doctor was making small talk about my job and my school history. I was just thinking, "Please get to the point." I could see the X-ray, and it was dark but full of shapes everywhere that looked like a cauliflower. I had no idea what it meant. Finally, I could see he was getting to the point.

He smiled at me and said, "I'm very, very sorry but we can't help you, you have a small percentage chance of recovery." He kept saying "I'm so sorry" all the time. I was just thinking, "Yeah sure you are." He showed me the X-ray. "This is a tumour," he said. "Tumour? Will I die?" I asked. I could see what he was referring to, it was huge and all over the place. He said it was so big that it could kill me any day if it were not removed or treated.

I just sat there looking around the room trying to get my head around it. "A tumour," I said. He said he was surprised I had not been showing symptoms a long time ago as it was one of the biggest, he had seen. Must have been growing for around 10 years he said. I said I had been telling my GP I had problems for years, but they wouldn't help me He said he was going to get me a bed ASAP and get me into surgery. I felt sick. I just said, "Wow, OK." What else can you say to that?

The doctor said that he would go off and organise a hospital bed at St George's for that night and asked if I wanted to stay with him while he was getting some things sorted. I said, "No thank you," and that I was fine. I refused to cry in front of him or anyone else for that matter. I just wanted him to go away so I could take in what he had said. The minute he walked away, I thought I was going to throw up. He went away for about 20 minutes which felt like an hour. I just remember thinking "Is this for real? I'll never see my family and friends. I'll never have children or grow old with someone."

My parents and Ian were in Australia and might not make it back to see me. How was I going to tell them on the phone? I went numb all over. I prayed for the strength to handle it, and I really hoped that I would go to heaven as I would see people again in the end, and that gave me some comfort. I wiped my eyes and just accepted it, and I wanted to make my last few days good ones with a smile on my face. I called Roland and told him what the doctor had said, and that I needed to go to St George's Hospital later. He said to come straight over to his house, and he would take me.

The doctor came back and gave me the details for my admission to St George's. He held my hand and said really slowly "Go and do what you need to do and then come back later, they'll be expecting you." I could see the doctor was not giving me any hope. I didn't really know what to say to him except "thank you for your help" I laughed at this as it was somewhat ironic.

It was 16:30 by the time I left the hospital. I walked to Roland's mum's house five minutes away from the hospital and rang the doorbell; I'd never known him to get to the door so quickly. He gave me a huge hug, and I burst into tears. I think I always deal with things OK on my own, but the second I see someone's face, I'm off again with the waterworks. When he hugged me it really made me realise the seriousness of what was happening. Roland looked at me and said that he thought that they had made a mistake, he said he couldn't explain why, but that the doctor had made a mistake. "It is not your time. God is in control," he said quietly, and I quickly agreed with him.

I went in and sat down. I needed to make some calls to see if people could see me before my operation.

Although I knew that Camilla, Becca and Emma wouldn't be able to make it I phoned them first. I wasn't sure how I was going to tell them. I called Camilla first as she had been calling me all day and keeping in touch. It broke my heart to tell her the news. I remember her crying, and her voice was so sad. I tried everything not to let her panic and to be very positive. Her mum had to take the phone off her because she broke down in a shop in Reading and I explained to Sylvia what had happened.

This was another time I knew God was with me because I wanted to cry so much, but I had God holding me up, and I was utterly calm. I called Becca but she was so relaxed, and I couldn't believe how easy it was to tell her. Later I found out Roland had called her already with a heads up so that she didn't get upset on the phone. She put on a pretty fantastic voice, and I was shocked at how easy she made it. I called Emma, but it went to answer the phone, and I didn't think it was appropriate to leave a message. I then called my parents in Australia, and Mum answered the phone. I tried to be really to the point, and I kept being positive, telling her God was in control. I knew they didn't believe in him, but he really was with me. Mum said they'd get back to the UK as soon as they could.

Mum said that I should call her sister, Anne, and she could speak to the hospital as she used to be a nurse and could understand all the hospital jargon. I did, and Anne said that she would be in the hospital first thing the next morning. I had the whole day in hospital on the 22nd May 2008, and my operation would be on the next day at 08:00. After finishing on the phone, Roland said that he had spoken to our Pastor and Sister Gill and to our friends Everton and Vanessa and that we would all meet at our Church to pray about the situation and for a miracle. First, we went to my house and met Vanessa and Everton there. They were in shock, but I just said we must not worry. We met Pastor and Sister Gill at the Church. They all placed their hands on me, and we asked for a miracle and that His will would be done.

Roland, Everton, Ness and I went to get some takeaway from a Chinese. I went home and collected all of my things. I had the best friend I could ever have with Roland; every time I would slightly doubt, he just made a joke to lighten the situation, and I would just laugh with him. I tidied the house up entirely and emptied all the bins. I think that was my obsessive-compulsive disorder (OCD) coming out. We went back to the hospital at 23:30 – we were very late, but I decided that if I was going to be having hospital food for a long time, I was getting my Chinese in first. We went to the hospital, and I remember my vision was getting bad again. I think the body can give up even if your heart hasn't. The night nurse said they were waiting for me. I knew that I was going to be there for a long time, so I didn't hurry, but I did apologise. I said goodbye to Everton, Ness and Roland and I got into my hospital bed. Surprisingly, I fell asleep very quickly.

I woke up early the next day hoping that my parents would get there before I went down into the theatre. I phoned my work and explained what was happening to HR and spoke to my friend Nirm to explain. She was really calm, even though it must have been a big shock. Nirm said that she would let everyone know and organise a card, she would start a collection and I said perhaps I would have to use the money for some nice wigs, as I was told my hair would be shaved.

Avoiding talk of the spectra of the worse outcome, we talked about when I would get out. We said we would go shopping when I came home and buy some funny wigs, perhaps blue or red. I never thought that I would have to ask for a wig as a present. I noticed that I had loads of missed calls from people at work, but I couldn't deal with talking to them. I would just let Nirm pass on the news. She really couldn't understand how I could be so calm. I explained that my faith was strong and that was all. I also phoned Camilla and Becca to talk to before the operation.

My Pastor came in with Sister Gill to see me and brought me a card called 'Footprints in the Sand'. I really love the quote, and I then heard Leona Lewis had brought a song out that was called 'Footprints in the Sand'. It was a song that just felt like it was written to encourage me, which it did. It was overwhelming how many people were all there for me. Aunty Anne came to see me and went to speak with the doctors to get a better idea of all the details. My cousins all came in to say hello or just called me. People were so lovely, but I could tell they didn't know what to say. I had never seen so many magazines in one place. I just smiled all the time because I was very content, and I felt that I knew I would be fine. I just wished everyone could have been as confident as I was. My parents called me in the late afternoon and said they had got to Kuala Lumpur and were hoping to get to me first thing Friday morning.

My surgeon, Dr Minhas, came to introduce himself to me and explained what was happening. He discussed potential risks, such as problems with balance, coordination, speech, vision, memory or muscle function, depending on which area of my brain was being operated upon. He said he would not know the extent until we were in surgery. I asked him not to take too much of my hair off if he could help it. I had just had my hair done, over the weekend. I laughed, but he didn't.

I said I had already sorted out a wig for later. He still didn't laugh. He said I had a very, very large tumour the size of a grapefruit and it would take two operations. He said it would take around seven to eight hours for each one and I would have to have the second operation later on. One downside was that I might lose my vision as the tumour was in a tricky place. I said "I trust you. God is in control, and he already told me things will be fine." He smiled with a doctor's smile, like "God? Oh yes, hmmm!!" I just grinned. I was totally confident. I didn't even spend time thinking about what would happen if I lost my sight or speech.

Everyone left my bedside, and I used the time to call Emma. I called and told her the situation and not to worry and I would see her after I had the operation. I know that she was worried and later on she told me how she broke down in tears. Luckily, she was staying at the house of a friend who was able to console her.

I woke up very early on Friday 23rd May 2008 and the doctors came in at 06:00 to give me the especially unattractive hospital nightgown and to fit me with my arm bracelets. It was all becoming very real, and I continued to pray for strength and that I would not be worried, as no matter what - I would be fine. I filled out all the paperwork for the operation, and they said they would be collecting me at 08:00.

20 minutes before I was due to go down for the surgery, the door swung open, and my parents came running into my room. "We're here!" They had come straight from Heathrow Airport. It really looked like a scene from a movie. Sort of went into slow-motion. I could see they were relieved, and so was I.

I told them St George's Hospital is one of the best neurosurgery units in the country and I hoped that fact would give some comfort to my family. I could see that they were worried and that made it very hard for me. Two orderlies came to take me down to the theatre. I was still trying to be strong, but then I saw my dad was crying. I knew that my family and friends had no idea whether or not I would even come back. I waved goodbye, smiled and said: "I'll see you soon." The surgical team were standing over my trolley now and talking to me. The next thing...I was out like a light.

OK! Go and grab a coffee or a toilet break. That was intense!!

10 Hours Later

I was in surgery for 10 hrs. The hospital had sent my parents' home, and they just waited by the phone for the hospital to say the operation was over. The phone never stopped ringing with family and friends; everyone wanted to know if there was any news. It must have been terrifying just waiting and waiting. They eventually gave up waiting and came up to the hospital because they were afraid of falling asleep and missing the call to say how it went. 10 hours later my parents were told the operation seemed to have gone well.

Now it was a waiting game until I woke up and they could assess the effects of the surgery. I was kept asleep in the intensive care unit for a further 24 hours. I know my parents and Becca came in every day, but I was never awake much. I would drift in and out of sleep. After three days I was taken into the high dependency unit for two weeks and then went to the regular ward for two days until I left on the 6th of June.

Fantastic news came from Dr Minhas. He told my parents he was able to remove a 10cm tumour in one go; I had an intraventricular meningioma. Only 2% of people ever get this type of tumour. I wouldn't need another operation! Dr Minhas told my parents the tumour was so big that when they removed it, my entire brain moved over. I didn't know the good news yet myself, but I was not worried at all. I knew God was in control and no matter what happened I would be ok. We would have to wait for the tests to come back, but Dr Minhas was sure the tumour was benign.

Intraventricular meningiomas are rare tumours. The origin of these tumours can be traced to embryological invagination of arachnoid cells into the choroid plexus. What a mouthful that is.

Intraventricular meningiomas are slow-growing tumours that can grow very large before detection. Although they are commonly seen in the lateral ventricles, they occur in the third and fourth ventricles as well. Intraventricular tumours cause headaches for some time as much as a recorded 16 years before detection of the tumour.

Headaches, intermittent or persistent, are the most common symptom.

The most common effect of surgery to remove an intraventricular meningioma is speech disturbance. Recovery can be difficult if there is a postoperative cerebrospinal fluid leak. Most people with this tumour have visual field deficit, disconnection syndrome, or speech and cognitive deficits.

A diagnosis must be established using MR imaging, and surgery requires planning to avoid eloquent area damage. Early control of the vascular supply to the tumour is critically important, and the tumour can usually be removed intact without damage to vital areas around the ventricles. No recurrences have been reported after complete excision.

That was what the doctors said, but everyone is different so it would just take time to see if I had disabilities. While I was in the land of Nod. I had some crazy dreams. I never knew if they were real or not. I had to ask my parents or Becca when I woke up.

I was only scared once with the dreams, and that was at the beginning at the operation I think, as I dreamt the anaesthetic didn't work and I hadn't fallen asleep yet, and no one had realised. I was going to be awake during the operation, and I was trying everything to tell someone, but I couldn't speak or move. It was a room full of other patients waiting to be operated, one after the other like a car wash because once you were locked in you couldn't move until after the process. I did panic a bit, and I was asking God to help me to relax. This was not for long, but it was quite horrifying. I then went to a completely different dream where I was feeling God's presence and that I had nothing to worry about because He was there the whole time just watching over me.

After the strange dream about the operation, I could see someone, which was similar to my uncle John, who came every time I was sleeping and stood with me no matter where I was. He never spoke, but I knew that God was sending a messenger to let me know He was there. At one time, I could see what looked like ghosts, the kind you see in the children's programmes. There was these floating ghost looking images all tied to crosses like the crucifixion. I just smiled because I knew that the Devil would love to use this kind of opportunity to scare me, as I was helpless. I am such a wimp usually, but I felt very comforted knowing God was with me.

In one shocking dream, I was sure that I had woken up during my operation; my body was like a hefty weight. I had no feeling; all I could do was move my eyes. It was strange, but it didn't hurt, it was just a little unnerving. I heard voices around me. To my surprise, I was told after leaving the hospital that I had been woken up in my operation, and that was a standard check on brain function and a test to see if I could say 'yes' or 'no', or just blink and look at them. I fell asleep very quickly, but it was a bizarre few minutes.

In the high dependency unit, I slept most of the time, only coming around now and then. I couldn't speak, but at that point, I thought that was because I was just tired. However, I was about to find out that my speech would be affected for a lot longer than a few days. I could understand what I was seeing but couldn't understand what people were saying to me. I tried to speak when I was asked questions, but it didn't come out right. The doctors explained that I knew what I was looking at, but when I tried to speak it was just jumbled up. They said my speech was going to be hard to recover, and they wouldn't know how much I had lost; only time would tell. I just smiled because even though I was talking rubbish then, I knew that God hadn't brought me that far to deny me a full recovery. I was just so confident, I wouldn't accept my disabilities.

I was pleased to see people even with my jumbled or non-existent speech. Becca would be there every day and sit with me, and I was so glad to see her. She would try to brush my hair a bit as I was looking like the Grinch. She would cut my fingernails as I was scratching my face without realising a lot. I was blessed to have such a great friend.

I remember Roland came in with Reka one day. They were flying to Hungary and came to say goodbye even though it wasn't visiting time. Roland was being his usual self, getting around the nurses. I smiled a lot and hoped people would know how thankful I was for them being there. I was more than happy for people to come and say hello. I would continue to smile and watch everyone else talking to each other. I didn't have a clue what they were saying. I would smile and then fall asleep. I wasn't the greatest conversationalist, to be honest!

It seems I had got into a bad habit of sleeping all day and staying awake all night. I remember the nurses coming around in the evening to wash me, and I was so out of it. I was embarrassed but had no coordination to say I didn't like it. I couldn't speak yet, let alone move properly. I had a night nurse who would give me a number of my medications. I had to take around 20 tablets, which were spread out over the day. I hated the night ones at around midnight. I didn't realise this was a procedure, and I was convinced my night nurse wanted to kill me as she was very heavy-handed. I remember thinking, "Step back lady, I'm a child of God".

I had to have injections all the time. All the needles hurt but they were not horrific, and by the last week I would just look away and say "Go for it but, can't you use my bum"? My arms were looking like pincushions and were multi-coloured. I hoped when I got out of hospital people didn't think I was taking recreational drugs.

My blood was taken every day, and when one of the nurses came in, I asked, "Will you be leaving some of that for me?" She never seemed to find my sense of humour funny. I can't imagine why not. I had another man from Poland who was giving me my antibiotics, and I asked him, "Can you change my arm as that one is a little sore?" He always looked really guilty. But, I guess it is better than, he smiles while I said it.

One of the downsides of having brain surgery is seizures, and I had my first one in the hospital. This bit will make you laugh, or cringe…. After the surgery, I had a head drain which was there to basically drain the brain fluid that had built up where the tumour was. I was always told I had to have the drain above my head so the brain fluid would go out properly. I couldn't get out of bed until that was off me. After a week I had the drain taken out, I could sit up and finally stand up.

This one is embarrassing, but I can laugh now, kind of, anyway. I had three drips in my arm, and I thought one of them was my food as I was never hungry. I was told they were worried I hadn't been eating and they wanted me to try. I looked at my three drip bags, and I said: "Hmmm, those three bags are my food and medication going in to keep everything in liquid form, right?" "No, they are just medication; you need to eat more to gain your strength." I'm like, "Oh boy, silly me!"

After eating some food, I soon needed the loo. I was given a bucket on the bed, and I was thinking, 'No way, that is messy, I wanted to try but I just couldn't as I was really not liking the idea. The nurse then pulled over a portable toilet. I know I hadn't eaten much, but I still seemed to need a number 2. (Yes, that's what I said, stop laughing boys and girls, stop hiding your faces behind your hands!).

I tried to get out of bed and stand up and tried to sit on the portable toilet, I didn't realise how weak I was, and my body was like a dead weight, and my arms were shaking. Next, I opened my eyes, and I was back in bed with a gas mask on my face feeling very sick and surrounded by nurses. I had my first seizure. My mum said I had had a Grand-Mal Seizure.

Oh great, I thought 'Hello I am 'THE POO GIRL WHO FITTED'.

It's just as well I have a good sense of humour. I was still determined to get up on my feet and go to the regular toilet. Slowly I was wobbling around the ward and leaning on the handles that were all around the rooms. I was very weak on my right side of the body and was told I would need physio to help with that and sensation and feeling was not really there.

Now that I could get around, I went to the toilet, and when I went in, I pulled the emergency cord instead of the flush. I suddenly heard an alarm and commotion outside the bathroom door. I didn't want to open the door as I realised what I had done. I slowly opened the door and just said 'Oops, my bad'.

My thought processes were interesting; I would call people by the wrong name or just didn't know their names at all. It would tire me out to talk as it took me a long time to say what I wanted to. I would call my dad "one of my parents", as I couldn't remember the word, Dad.

I started to have more family visitors and tried hard to think and speak. I told my grandparents who are both very short, more like 5'4''ish, that they would never have the same problem that my feet were having. My feet were always sticking out the bed. I had to wear lots of socks to make up for the short mattress, and they seemed to feel really cold all the time and never warmed up. They do give you the socks in hospital, but for some reason one of the nurses rolled mine down to my ankle and although I didn't feel it until afterwards, getting out the hospital the hospital socks have left a scar on both ankles where it cut my blood circulation. I see them as a reminder that I'm still walking and alive.

My parents and my grandparents and Becca had come in every day. I asked my mum what the history was behind my nickname Wookie, which my grandad kept calling me. She said my uncle Chris (one of my Godfathers) was a Star Wars fanatic and didn't like my dad's nickname for me, Clairey-Cluey. Chris said "Hmm, 'Cluey' rhymes with 'Chewy', which is Chewbacca's nickname in Star Wars. Chewy is a Wookie Bear…I think you should be called Wookie," and the name stuck.

My mum said I had something like 30 texts from people on my mobile while I was in the hospital. I couldn't read them, they didn't make sense to me. I would have to wait for somebody to read them too me. My Pastor and Sister Gill came in to see me again and pray for my situation. They were so supportive of me.

I was able to watch the TV or listen to some music; finally, I couldn't take in what was happening, but I just liked the distraction from the ward I was in. Hospitals have gone up in the world with electronics. You can do anything from your bed without asking for help. You must pay for the TV, but it was a small price to pay instead of hearing what everyone is doing around you in the ward. The ward itself is like watching the program

Casualty, but it gets depressing after a while, watching sick people.

Finally, about four days before leaving the hospital I was able to have a bath. I couldn't get water on my scar as it needed to stay dry. It was still the most beautiful bath I had ever had. I didn't want to get out. I hated the whole being bathed in my bed every day by different nurses. On the 2nd of June, I was moved to another room. It was nice being taken out of the high dependency unit and have all the machines taken away. Now I was just waiting to be sent home.

I was sharing a ward with six other ladies now. They were all there for different head operations. One lady opposite me was in for the same reason as myself. She was Greek and very loud but lovely. Her family would come and see her all the time. Another lady was next to me and was there for a tumour that they could not help her with. She would die at some point within a year she was told, and she was only about 50. She was such a sweet lady, but I could see she was scared. I would just pray for her a lot that she would not suffer.

Time to Go Home

On the 6th of June, the doctor came in to say I could go home. He gave me a huge box full of tablets. I looked like a walking chemist. He explained a few things to my parents and me. I wasn't really paying attention, and I didn't really take in what they had said. Looking back now, it was information I wish I'd listened to. Then it wouldn't have been such a shock later, having to wait for my rehabilitation.

The doctor said I would have short- and long-term effects. He noted that swelling of the brain can cause weakness, poor balance and coordination, personality changes, speech problems and fits. I now had lost my peripheral vision, and I would need to hand my drivers license to the DVLA. He said the symptoms would usually lessen or disappear as I recover. He said I needed to be patient as this process could take months after such an extensive operation. Because of the position of the tumour, I might have long-term problems with speech or with the weakness of an arm or leg. But with effort and help from physiotherapists, speech therapists and other rehabilitation specialists, the doctor was confident that I would get a lot better.

My rehabilitation would start as soon as I could move around more. I was told not to expect instant results! I would gradually be able to do more and more for myself. I was warned that I might never quite recover the same level of fitness as before my illness, but that my condition would improve. I would need time to regain my energy.

I remember standing up all ready to go home. It was so pleasant to wear my shoes again although I kept saying "I have my feet on" instead of shoes. I brushed my hair very carefully and tried not to get upset as I was finally going home. 17 days ago, there had been a question over my life, and I just kept holding onto God the whole time. He indeed is astounding to me.

I wobbled out of the hospital. My legs were like boulders – they felt as though I'd just run a marathon. It didn't matter how much I wanted to walk faster out the door, I couldn't. I kept looking at my hands in amazement because they had finally stopped shaking after two years. I was very spaced out, but I was happy to breathe fresh air rather than the hospital wards. I put my thoughts and situation into God's hands and was very strong in hospital, but when we were driving out of the car park, it dawned on me that people didn't think I was coming back. I realised how much God took care of my emotions in the hospital.

As I got home, I started feeling very sick, the kind of feeling that sits in the pit of your tummy. I was determined not to cry because I was happy, but I was emotional. It was very overwhelming how much mail I had when I walked into the house. I had told my parents not to bring me any cards or presents as I didn't want to feel like I was ill. I was on a mission to get up and out. I could tell from messages in the cards people were anxious about how extreme my situation was, and that was something I hadn't wanted to see before but afterwards, it was very very humbling how caring people are. My company had sent the biggest bunch of flowers I had ever seen, and the vase was gorgeous. I went upstairs, very slowly I might add as I was very weak, and my balance was off. I went to my room, and it was bizarre being there, even though everything was as I left it.

I looked around; everything was as I had left it. I read through all my cards and people were so lovely, even people I hardly knew had sent cards. One of my best presents was that my company said I had been made permanent two weeks before getting back home. I was so happy because, I just felt so grateful, and it was a massive weight off my shoulders as I had finished my probation a few days before I went into the hospital. I thanked God for the news. It felt like everything was going to be ok like God had put his hand on me, and everything was calm. I don't mean the situation, but my mindset was strong.

My mum said I was going to be off work getting better for some time and I should find things to do. That was hard to deal with, I thought I would be off for a few weeks but, I never imagined I would be off for six months. Most people would say how cool to have that time off, but I didn't know how not to work. It seemed like the next part of my life was going to be harder still. I felt I'd won the battle but still needed to win the war.

The minute I got home I called Camilla who I hadn't spoken to since just before my operation. I tried to make some witty comment, but I found speaking hard, and nothing would come out right. She wasn't around, so I left a jumbled-up voicemail to say, "Hi guess who." She called back in about two minutes. My speech was not good, It was difficult on the phone, so I let Camilla do all the talking which made a change as I am usually the one with the motor mouth.

When I looked in the mirror for the first time in a long time, I noticed my pupils were huge, and I couldn't see the iris in my eyes. It looked weird. The doctor had said my pupils would get back to normal after a week or two. I then looked at my scar. It looked like Frankenstein was looking in the mirror. I was not liking the view.
I then realised I couldn't see clearly. I couldn't see my reflection fully in the mirror. I just asked God to give me the strength to stop focusing on my appearance.

The next thing I wanted to do was have a nice hot shower with some privacy, not being watched by nurses' eagle eyes. Just to be sure I didn't fall over Mum stayed nearby. I was told not to put the shower directly on where my incision was for about two months.

Camilla rushed down to see me on the second weekend. It was nice to see her. We were both trying not to get emotional over what had happened. We just laughed at things to brush off the uneasy elephant in the room, being my crazy last 2 weeks. I couldn't talk too much about it as it was hard. I was happy to see her.

I was very thankful to be home, but things were different, and I was finding it hard to be patient. My good friend Naomi from college came over on the second day bought me a huge bunch of helium balloons saying get well soon. I had never seen so many balloons in one place, it was such a pleasant surprise, and I was pleased to make use of them when they were going down. I could suck out the helium and have conversations on the phone with friends. It's the little things that made me giggle; OK, OK, I know, but give me a break – I didn't get out much! And I really needed a laugh. Mentioning laughing, one other thing that was amusing was I always seemed to leave my flies down even when I was putting my jeans on in the morning. Then later in the day I'd go to the loo and realise they were open. I'd see what I'd done and laugh and then forget to do them up again! There were and still are a few mind blocks, but that one I sorted out quickly with just using stretchy trousers without zips.

Sent to Rehab.

In mid-July 2008 I started with a private speech tutor who helped me for three weeks, getting me ready for attending the NHS Neuro-rehabilitation centre in Croydon. She explained what had happened to my speech and that I should be able to have most of it back, but it depended on how affected the brain had been. It may never be perfect, but with strategies, I could cope. She said that usually words and memory are all stored, in the brain, like a filing system. When we want to remember something or speak, we automatically go to the right file to get it. During the operation, all these files had been thrown up in the air and had become entirely disorganised, with the result that it takes longer to find the right file.

After three weeks I was finally able to start my rehabilitation programme for speech and language therapy, physiotherapy, occupational therapy and relaxation therapy. Relaxation and occupational therapy were to help me cope with everyday things and get me ready to return to work. The first thing I thought when I heard the word 'rehab.' was Amy Winehouse or Britney Spears. I guess I thought rehab was for people with bad habits.

When I arrived, I didn't like it. I didn't want help from people, I was fine. I didn't need to feel needy. It was the first time I would be talking to people other than friends and family. I remember on the first day I went to meet my new speech and language teacher Michelle. She seemed nice and was very welcoming. I had to answer a bunch of questions about myself and what had changed for me after the operation. She said, right at the beginning, "Please don't worry if you cry at this part, as we understand it is a tough subject to talk about." I just smiled and said, "No, no, that's fine, I'm fine with everything." Within minutes I had burst into tears. There went my chilled-out look, right out the window. It brought everything to my attention, about what had happened and how extreme my situation was. It was highlighting all the disabilities I now had. That was only the first day at rehab, and I wasn't comfortable with things at all!

I then had my physiotherapy with Elaine the next day. She was gentle but very firm which I liked because I knew she would get my body sorted out. She had to do an assessment to see what parts were causing a problem. The evaluation showed I was very, very weak on my right side and that my balance was awful. Because I had lost vision out of the right corner of the eye, it took me a long time to adjust my peripheral sight. I would get tired very quickly. Elaine would say it wasn't about doing things for hours, it was about doing a small bit each day because I needed to take it easy. My rehab classes were all about long sessions with lots of breaks in between. Elaine felt I would benefit from doing Pilates. It's an excellent fitness programme that you can push yourself at, at any level. Anyone, at any age, could do this. It all depends on your own level of fitness.

My next session was occupational therapy. I met Susie, and she explained that she would be the person to talk with my HR department to plan a back-to-work strategy. I then had to do some questionnaires to see where my weaknesses were. She asked me what my most important goal at rehabilitation was. I said I wanted to get back to work as soon as I could and wanted to get back to my normal life. She was pleased with my determination, but she said I needed to understand I would be in rehab for three months, and I would not be able to rush back to my old life. That was another tough conversation. I felt helpless but I was determined to get back to my life, and I knew God had already brought about one miracle in my life. In Matthew 19:26 it says, "with man this is impossible, but with God all things are possible". I just kept this with me. I wasn't going to give up. I would just keep praying and reminding myself that everyone is on this earth for a reason. It was up to me to find out what that reason is and to be the best at it. God had done his part for me, now it was my turn to do mine!

During my rehabilitation that I decided to start turning my diary into a book. It was a way of keeping me busy. I didn't want to feel sorry for myself. I needed to stay positive, and the book would remind me that I had come a long way and I wasn't about to give up now.

I started relaxation classes in the last week at rehab. I was always the youngest person in rehab but, I met many great people who were mainly there after having a stroke.

I did meet one lady, and she had the same tumour as I did, except when she had her operation they had to go through a different part of the brain. They must make a choice about where they go in to get the tumour out. I knew that was a choice they had had to make during my operation and that the decision was made to give the best chance of saving my abilities, both physically and mentally. With the other lady, they went through a different part of the brain. She had substantially lost her movement and needed a cane to walk.

One of the other things I was doing, to help my speech and memory, was singing. One of my passions in life is singing, but after my operation, I couldn't anymore. I could hum to a tune, but when I opened my mouth, no words came out or if they did they were wrong. I have also always played the piano, and strangely I could still play that but not sing. I have never been able to read music and just play by ear. I couldn't believe I could again do it.

Now that I had been home for two months, lots of people were asking me to meet up, but, it was hard for me. My medication was making me so hot all 24/7. My skin was glowing with sweat. It sounds as gross as it was, I was very uncomfortable leaving the house. I found everywhere with more than one person talking was overwhelming. Small crowds were beginning to sound like a football match to me. I was knocking into things as I couldn't see clearly. I was turning down offers to meet up.

I just sat in the garden most days as it was still lovely and warm outside. My mum bought me a DS with the Brain Training game. Just to show you how poor my memory was: it took me three months to get my brain age score down from 80 to 30.

I was then given an appointment for my scan. The first scan was strange because you usually have a scan and then end up with an illness, but I was just reminded all the time about what had happened when what I really wanted was to forget it, put it behind me and go back to my life. I remember the scan on the 19th June was quick and my parents and Becca came with me. We left and I was falling asleep in the car, as always, I was ready for bed.

I was called the next day, from the hospital, which was not normal, and Dr Minhas said he had a concern with my scan. He said I had some bleeding in the brain and I may need to have a drain put in. This could mean another operation. I was so scared of going back in again. I needed encouragement, I needed prayers, and I sent a text to my Pastor and Sister Gill and some other close friends from Church and asked for their prayers. I didn't go into details, but I was freaking out, and I couldn't control it. It's like stubbing your toe, only 10 times worse. You don't want to do it the first time, and you certainly wouldn't want to do it again.

I went to see Dr Minhas. Becca and my parents were with me. When I got there, I went straight to the toilet. Becca came with me, and I couldn't stop shaking. It was horrible, and I couldn't make it stop. Becca just gave me a hug and told me to take deep breaths and relax. I tried to remind myself God was there, but I was still so nervous. Eventually, I managed to calm down and splashed some water on my face. I just prayed to God I could get through the meeting and could crack-up afterwards. We went in, and Dr Minhas said he wasn't going to go on too much, but the scan had shown I had some bleeding in the brain and he was hoping some steroids would stop it. If not, I would have an operation to drain the blood and the fluid. I left the room, and I was not sure how to feel. I was certain God my back, and I just needed to relax. I was exhausted when we got home, I was numb all over. I just asked for more prayers from my Church.

I started the two-week course of steroids in the morning, and over the next two weeks, I became a recluse at home, as though it was some sort of cocoon that would keep any harm from befalling me. I just went to rehabilitation for a few hours every day and then came straight home. I didn't want to speak to anyone, as I knew I was getting aggressive. I didn't want to behave that way, so I just kept to myself; I was crying at the smallest thing and couldn't control it. My teachers said they could see a significant shift in my behaviour and demeanour and said I should check with my doctor. I went to the doctor, who noted that mood swings were very normal with the steroids I was on. I could be happy or sad. I was not in the most fabulous place, but my doctor said I would be finished soon. Once I was off the steroids, I went back to myself. It was crazy to think some tablets that help, radically change your personality.

Good news came on the 5th of September as, after another CT Scan, Dr Minhas called me and said that the blood had gone, and the steroids had worked. I was to come back in November as there was still some fluid although the bleeding had gone, which was great. I went again on the 2nd of November for another scan. I didn't realise that I was going to have an MRI which was very scary. I saw all the same people I had seen there six months earlier, and that was quite hard. I was not fazed by the scans, I was so used to them. I just didn't realise I was going to have an MRI. I was happy to leave that day.

I called Dr Minhas, to see if the results were good. I asked if I could travel now and he said YES, he said that the fluid had all but gone now and he would be writing to my GP to reduce my medication. He would send a letter out with an appointment to see him in December.

I was so happy with the news. My friend Emma was back in London from Dubai which is where she lives now with her fiancé. We were pleased with the good news from Dr Minhas, and she suggested I should go back with her to Dubai for a week. I said "Great!" and we booked a ticket the next day for a week of relaxation and getting me out of the house and back into life! I was nervous to fly as I had heard that I may have trouble with cabin pressure on the plane. That the fluid in my head could get worse.

We arrived at Terminal 5 and went to the First-Class area because Emma was a corporate cardholder. I was thrilled to take advantage of all the free food, magazines, drinks and more food. We were so relaxed we didn't realise that our plane was about to leave. We had to rush through the terminal to our departure gate.

We got there very out of breath. The ladies there gave us a very disapproving look, telling us severely that they were just about to take our bags back off the plane. Then Emma did the funniest thing, and any nervous feelings I had about flying and the cabin pressure on the plane disappeared. She hobbled up to the counter and said, "Ow my leg, owww!" I was trying so hard not to laugh. She continued to wobble on to the plane with noises like "Ouch!" and "Ooh". We got on the plane and could see everyone else was already seated. We looked at each other and just burst out laughing. The air hostess was clearly trying not to laugh with us and said, "No problem girls." We flew off, and I spent so much time laughing and catching my breath that I didn't have a second to worry about flying or how the pressure in the cabin might affect me. We had a relaxing week, and I was so happy I had gone there. I felt like my life was coming back and I was looking forward to Christmas and New Year's Eve on its way.

Christmas and New Year's Eve came and went. I had caught the nasty flu. I couldn't hold any food down. I was determined not to let it stop me from going back to work in January. I went to the hospital for a check-up. I had to see a different surgeon instead of Dr Minhas. I was trying to stay positive, but the new surgeon seemed so unhelpful. I was expecting to be told I could come off the seizure tablets and that I would be able to drive again if my eyes had got better. I didn't expect him to say I was going to be on my pills forever! The surgeon was so happy about the job they had done with y operation and less concerned, it seemed, with my getting back to a normal life.

It had been a very long wait, but I finally went to get my eyes tested at the hospital the next day. I was told I was on the borderline of having enough vision to drive again and getting my license back. I would need to have the test again in May 2010. Suddenly things were becoming disappointing. I prepared myself for more disappointment and once again put my trust in God.

Back to Work

At the end of January 2009, I could finally start back at work. I knew I had some things still to sort out with the hospital, but I was well enough to go back to work. I seemed to be settled on my tablets, I was on 1000mg Tegretol. I had no seizures since in the hospital.

It was great seeing everyone in the office. They were so welcoming. For the time that I was away from work having surgery and rehabilitation, a 'temp' had taken on my role. Now it was her having to teach me my own job. The temp would continue to work with me until I was back full time which would not be for at least 6 weeks. It took a lot of pressure off me.

In the evening I spoke to Camilla on the phone. I let her do all the talking because I was muddling up my words, I was exhausted. I said I would get an early night and would call her back the following day. Soon later, I was fast asleep in bed.

On Thursday the 16th of January, I was abruptly awoken by my mobile phone ringing loudly. It was Camilla calling me back. The ring really shocked me. My parents were out of the house. I should have ignored the phone and gone back to sleep, but I never expected what was about to happen actually happen.

I was trying not to butt in on the conversation and tried to ignore the sick feeling in my stomach and this weird feeling of exhaustion that had come over me. I was listening to Camilla, but I felt faint. I knew I should end the call, but I thought it was better to have somebody on the phone because I could feel that something was happening. I was trying to speak, but I was just mumbling. I told her not to worry but to call my mum or 999 because something was happening. This was the first seizure I had really been aware of, and I didn't know the protocol! I was gasping for breath. I tried to lie in the recovery position, hoping that was the right thing to do. I didn't know much about seizures. I was worried about the things I had seen on the TV about people chewing or swallowing their tongue. I could hear Camilla saying she would get help and that she was going to stay on the phone with me. I could feel my neck arching back. I was so frightened.

I woke up and wasn't sure why I was lying on the floor. I very realised what had happened. I could hear people shouting through the letterbox downstairs. I thought they were trying to break into my house, I was so disorientated. I crawled to my parents' on-suite bathroom and shut the door. I lay on the floor feeling horrible and sick. For some reason, I couldn't lock the door. My whole body was in shock, and my arms and hands wouldn't do anything even though I had just crawled there. I do believe that when a person is terrified, they find strength from somewhere.

Now I could move more, I just took a deep breath and thought, "I'll be fine, God, please protect me." I decided to go downstairs, and if I needed to, I would hurl myself out of the front door with all my might.

To my surprise, it was an ambulance team at the door. I was so glad to see them but scared at the same time. I couldn't speak very well, and I was in a real daze. They wanted to take me back to the hospital to be checked me out. They asked for the best number, and I gave my mum's. I was like jelly. One of the ambulance ladies called my mum from my mobile. I could imagine what a shock that was for her. She was going to get to the hospital as soon as she could and meet me there.

On the way to the hospital, three things were going through my mind. First, was I going to lose my license forever (how silly is that? As if that was the most important thing). The second thing was the whole sitting sideways in the ambulance was not a good feeling, and I hoped I would not be sick. The third thing was the question – am I going to have seizures forever? I had my priorities, right, didn't I?

I arrived at the hospital, and they checked my blood pressure, and I had to have a cannula and cardio-vascular examination. My mum turned up soon after me with my stuff, in case I had to stay overnight. I was so out of it. But again, I was very calm and just knew God was still giving me strength, I was allowed home very quickly after my blood tests came back fine. The feeling was that maybe my tablets were not strong enough. "Oh great," I was thinking. That was all I needed. I remember asking God if I could "have a break please". I got home and fell asleep next to Mum, I didn't want to be alone.

I went back to the doctor on Monday, and she signed me off work AGAIN!! I couldn't believe I only made it back to work for one day. They said I needed to have more blood tests and get my seizure tablets under control. I was not myself for another few weeks. Every time I stood up, I was very disorientated. I was so paranoid I would have another seizure. I started to investigate all the details about having seizures. I hated the word, and I felt sick thinking about it. I thought I was going to have to sell my car for sure and lose my license. I just prayed for God to comfort me and give me the strength to be positive.

I then booked an appointment to meet my neurologist and discuss what happened. He said my seizure would have been because my medication was not strong enough. I would need to gradually raise the dosage and keep having a blood test to see which dosage was the best for me and to stop any seizure. He said until I had the right level I may still have seizures. Well, there went my confidence out the window.

I was feeling really low about the situation. I just went into a cocoon; my bedroom was my safe place. I just wanted to get better and go back to my life.

On Friday 20th February I woke up early to have another blood test at the doctor's and to check my tablets levels were working well enough to allow me to go back to work. I would have to wait a few days to get the results. I was feeling a lot better physically. I was very nervous about going back to work as the last month had been a real set back and had knocked my confidence massively.

I received the blood test results on Wednesday 25th February. My results showed my current tablets were still not doing enough for me and I had to go back up even more. A week later the doctor said my levels were better. So, ones again I went back to work again. This time I was very nervous about having a seizure on the tube or bus or in my office.

I was hoping that I had had the last seizure now and never again. Although my body was well, my mind was now not well, I had lost confidence in myself. I was paranoid about having a seizure.

My first week back at work went well, other than the tiredness. February came and went, and I was happy being back to work but I had no social life except text messages from friends. I didn't want to over-do-it and then have a seizure. I had associated my last two seizures because I was exhausted and that is when it seems to happen.

Confidence Booster

While I was at home on my days off work, I was looking at things to do, I saw on Facebook there was a section you could talk to people from around the world. I was not very savvy at online forums. However, it was something to do.

Unexpectedly for me, I did meet somebody. A Corporal in the British Army. I had never met somebody in the military before. I found it interesting to hear about his last tour and what his role was. I never thought anything would come from our conversations. Bit by bit we got to know each other. He had mentioned that his mother had epilepsy and that really took a massive weight off my shoulders as he could understand what can happen with seizures. It was almost too good to be true. I had been so nervous about telling people about my brain tumour and the seizures, I was embarrassed to talk about it as I felt like people would treat me differently, do that nodding thing. The one where they tilt their head to the side and say "oh yes I see" – when they more than likely don't see at all.

By the end of March, we decided to meet up. His barracks were close to my friend Naomi in Chatham. I set up to stay at her house and then go for drinks with the corporal nearby. I had never ever met somebody through the internet, and I had my back up in place – Naomi and her husband Andy and their dogs, in case anything happened. I am such a drama queen but better be safe than sorry.

I met him on April 18th, 2009. I was so nervous about my seizures because knowing my luck I would have one while I was with him. The weekend went well, and we got on great. There were no seizures, and I had a new boyfriend!

The following week was going well at work, and I was coping with the travel to and from London. I had one of my days off and decided to tidy up the house and change the beds. I had been fine all week and had no problems on the commute home. But suddenly while changing the beds, I felt dizzy, hot and had a nasty metal taste in my mouth. I realised I was going to have another seizure. I was so frustrated because there was nothing, I could do about it. I called my mum who was downstairs at the top of my voice: "It is happening again!" "I'll be fine." The next thing I knew there were two ambulance people in my room. I was taken to the hospital to be checked over. They were happy to send me home after a few tests and told me to tell my GP about what had happened.

We went home, and I was exhausted. Back to my bed, I went and just wanted to forget about the day. I was so disappointed in myself. It must have been scary for Mum; she hadn't seen me have a grand mal seizure before. My Boyfriend said he would still be over the next day to give me some TLC.

I felt better after the weekend and went back to work. I was fatigued nevertheless, was determined to get through it. As Friday came and I had had a whole week with no drama I planned for my boyfriend and me to see my friends who lived a couple of hours from me. We went via train, and things were going well and lots of laughs and talking about life in general until I realised that I was feeling very unwell and felt as though I was going to have another seizure. I said I needed to go. We left, and my friend kindly offered to drive us back home. I was so grateful but once again, embarrassed. I felt like a child. They all said it was no problem, but I couldn't help feeling like a burden. I slept through the journey back and went straight to bed.

After the weekend I went back to work. I was so nervous but determined to get on with things. I was slowly building my confidence back up now that I was out and about a lot more. My boyfriend was giving me that extra confidence to push myself even if he didn't know it at the time.

On Thursday 7th May I went to my doctors to ask if it was normal the feelings I was having. Getting faint, disorientated and getting auras. After a blood test, my doctors and my neurosurgeon said I was being given the wrong seizure tablets by my GP. There is two types of Tegretol and mine had been mixed up which explained everything. I was furious about it, but I was also happy to get myself on the correct tablets and stop any aura's or seizure-like feelings. It is crazy when you put your life into the doctor's hands only to find they make mistakes too!

I needed to relax for the rest of the week in case I had a seizure while I adjusted my medication. I decided to stay at my boyfriend's house at his barracks instead of mine. I packed a bag and headed to Chatham. I just needed to keep calm and stay strong until I got to his barracks. It took me just over an hour on the train, but it felt like three hours.

The tablets were given a terrible side-effect. It was horrible. It was like I was being electrified which only lasted a second, but all I could think about was 'Here comes a seizure'. I shouldn't have gone, sometimes being stubborn is also silly. I finally got to Chatham station and got to the barracks. We just watched films and TV all night with ice cream and sweets. Very healthy, I know! I was ok throughout the night, and the terrible feelings had not come back. The following day we just carried on watching films. We were not planning to go anyway.

Then I was getting a funny shaky tingling feeling in my body. I was keeping positive that the feeling would pass. I was trying to relax, but then things got weird. I was shaking all over, and I couldn't open my eyes. I was lying there and thinking "God if there is any way you could intervene right now, I would really appreciate it." I didn't want to have a full-on seizure in front of the corporal. The last thing I needed was to start vibrating on the floor looking deformed and pee my pants. Nobody ever tells you that bit about seizures. I just wanted to go home, I wasn't in the right state of mind to get the train along, and my boyfriend only had a motorbike. On this occasion, both were not suitable. I just had one other choice, I called up my parents and told them what was happening, they were happy to pick me up.

I spent the weekend resting and building my strength back up. I knew what was happening with my body, so I didn't need to go to the hospital this time. I was determined to get through it and get back to work on

Monday. Thankfully I was feeling better and the whole week went by with no more weird episodes. I was still drained, but I was able to do easy tasks and was still only working part-time.

One of the weekends in July when I was staying at my boyfriend's barracks, I had planned to meet my work friends Amanda and Clare in Chatham. It was my first big night out since my surgery. Up until then I was way too tired and couldn't cope with crowds and noise. I was still on medication, so there was no alcohol for me. Sometimes it helps to have a drink to relax but, this wasn't an option for me.

So, on Saturday, I went to meet my friends, and my boyfriend went out with his army mates. It was nice to go out, but it was the first time, going on a full-on night. At first, I was struggling with the noise and lights in the bars but, I was determined to stay out and enjoy myself.

I loved being out. We bumped into corporal and his friends, and they were really drunk. I didn't mind, but I was a little embarrassed as this was the first time, he had met my friends properly. I had a great time with the girls, and I was not making a fuss over Corporal. He was very drunk and started talking to every girl in the bar. The girls were asking if I was OK with it as he was being very disrespectful but, for some reason, I didn't care. I just switched off and knew that even though he was a great friend he was not the one for me. The girls went in a taxi home, and I carried Corporal home to his place. I got him to bed, and he was out for the count. I was lying in bed and was wondering how I would tell him we should just be friends? I think it was just too soon for me to meet somebody.

The next day Corporal managed to get up and said he didn't remember much from the night before which made me laugh, but something told me that that's the way he was and that he clearly liked the attention he was getting from girls. We went to the army school he worked in first thing. It was not really a school, it was more an instructor's school for the army. It was really interesting finding out what he did. I met his colleagues and friends. They were very easy to talk to. I was starting to feel tired, and I knew that was the combined effect of my tablets and being out the night before. I just couldn't cope with the tiredness. As much as I wanted a night out, I knew I would be paying for it for a few days afterwards. I called Camilla to distract attention away from the fact that I was not talking to Corporal or the others. I told her I felt I would have to break up with Corporal, but I couldn't as we were booked to go to Australia in August. I stuffed a packet of nuts in my mouth and drank a lot of water. They had a barbecue, and I was straight up, first in the queue. It was the best burger ever, or was that because I was so hungry?

I went back to work the next Monday and just concentrated on my job, trying not to make a huge deal of the weekend. Corporal phoned me in the week and said his mum would need to have a skin graft. I felt sick for him. It is weird because I never met her, but I wouldn't put that on anyone. It is very scary and stressful for a person. It was definitely not the time to say we should just be friends. I know cancer and sickness is always with us in the world but when you have suffered from something it gives you a deep empathy with people's suffering.

I spent the next week working hard again, and the tablets seemed finally to be settling down. Three weeks later we were ready to go to Sydney. I was so excited about seeing Ian, and I was going to meet his new girlfriend, Phoebe. The flight to Sydney completely wiped me out, and I had really bad jetlag. It was so great to see Ian, but no matter how much I wanted to enjoy being with him, I was too tired. My body was aching all the time. We kept busy, and I started to think that going away had possibly been a bad idea. I wasn't ready. I think that was my fault because I wanted Corporal to see as much as he could in case he never came back to Sydney. I had been many times before.

Ian and Corporal got on well which was great, and I got on really well with Phoebe. Ian was a great host. He got us doing LOADS, thanks, Ian. We went on a road trip to lots of beautiful places. My tiredness was starting to show. I was getting crabby, and the smallest thing was annoying me. I kept it inside all holiday as I didn't want to argue or cause a scene that would ruin the atmosphere, but I think that was a bad idea. Right near the end of the trip I just couldn't cope with the tiredness and the jetlag any more. I was boiling over with frustration. I used my hairdryer, and it blew up! I laugh about it now but at the time my heart was beating so fast, and the incident really shocked me. I was scared because I was worried that something like that would trigger a seizure. I just wanted to scream from exhaustion, it was as though my hairdryer had felt the force of my frustration and simply blew up!

We got back to England and sitting beside him on the plane, even though we had had a lovely holiday, I knew my boyfriend, and I were over.

One morning, back at work, my colleague friend Louise found me on the bathroom floor feeling very unwell. I had fainted trying to splash my face with some water. I was so glad it was her that found me. The friendships I made at Petro-Canada were indeed a blessing. I was sent home and told that I just needed to take it easy and stop trying to be Superwoman! I wanted help with my tiredness and bought a treadmill to get fitter and to give me more strength in myself. I was using a Pilates video. I found it great to build me up without exhausting me. I was determined to get strong. I genuinely enjoy my fitness now. At least I know if I go out and about with my brother again, I will keep up, as I will have more strength.

By November 2009 I was feeling a lot better. I went to Dubai to see Emma and George for a week. I had a fantastic holiday, and it was obvious that at last, I was getting stronger physically and mentally. We did so many things, and I coped.

When I got back to work, I was made redundant. My company had merged with another oil and gas company, and they were closing down the London office in December 2009. I had known for months, so it wasn't a shock. I was looking forward to using some of the redundancy money and starting a new chapter of my life.

Time to Try Again

New year, new start – again lol. In December my friend Reka said she wanted to go to Thailand and being a spontaneous person (especially when travel is on offer), I said I'd go with her if she liked. I was able to use some of my redundancy money, and she was more than happy for us to go together. The next day we booked the holiday. We had two months to prepare, so I needed to work on my fitness. I don't mean fit for the sunbathing and looking trimmed, but I needed to work on my stamina so I could cope with a long and active holiday. It would be nice to spend March away as we both had birthdays coming up and we could celebrate them there. I was nervous, wondering if I would be feeling better by then but I hoped I would be fine. I didn't want to miss opportunities for going away or for getting a good job. I yearned to do something spontaneous, out of the ordinary. Thailand was a big challenge.

In January I was desperate to get off my seizure tablets because I was sure they were making me more tired than ever. I knew that Clobazam and Tegretol needed to be at the right level – not too high or too low. My fatigue started to get ridiculous again, and I was falling asleep every day, and at every opportunity, I had to lay my head down. I wanted to see my seizure doctor and see if he could help. I had only a month or two until I was due to jet off to Thailand.

Then I started having really strange feeling that I could have a seizure any time. I was 26 and falling apart again. I very quickly got an appointment with my seizure doctor, Doctor von Oertzen, who said they would lower my dosage from 1000 to 800mg as the dosage I was on was higher than I needed to be on. If that worked then great, but if not, he would have to think of another plan of action. I would have to wait for four/five weeks to benefit from the change in dosage.

I was getting worse and worse every day. My body was just shaking all the time and making me feel so sick. I was really scared I would have a seizure and every jolt in my body made me think it was the start of one.

I knew I was not ready to work yet as things were so unstable, but I was called by an agency that I had dealt with in the past, and they said they had a great job doing the same type of work as I had done before with the same pay. I thought it was unlikely I would get it as I was looking rough and could quite possibly be sick at any time. Through a determination not to give up on myself, I went to the interview. When I woke up on the day of the interview I felt awful, and I was not sure if I should go, but my dad said if I wanted, he would come with me and wait in the coffee shop opposite the offices. It was right by Regent Street and a lovely area for shopping fans. I went into the company and sat waiting. The feeling of electricity coursing through me would not go away. I had taken up my dad's offer to come with me, and so I could go straight home after the interview. I was so grateful for my parents' support. The interview went surprisingly well. I went home and went straight to bed, glad it was over.

The next day I had three missed calls from the agency. When I called them back, they offered me the job! Praise God, that was just the ego boost I needed. I don't know how I got it, but I guess my résumé was perfect for the job they were offering. The money was very tempting too, but every jolt that went through my body was just another reminder to say, "don't take it, you won't be able to do it". I was so very flattered, and I really wanted to take it. But I had to make the right decision, for me and for them, and I declined their offer later that day. They tried to offer me more money, but on this occasion, I knew I just would not be able to give them what they deserved and reluctantly I had to say goodbye to the opportunity.

I knew that I had to put my health first now. I had to get a more practical and achievable role while I got all my dosages sorted.

I went straight down to the doctors the next day. They said my blood test results showed that my dose of Tegretol was wrong and that led to my being sick. It took me two months to get the wrong tablets out of my system. I was angry with my doctor for making such a big mistake. The tablets come in two types, and they are identical in appearance, but if you read the boxes carefully, they have one small difference that makes a big difference to the patient, which my GP should know. After spending two months feeling unwell, I was back on track with the right medication.

On Monday 22nd February I went to see Dr von Oertzen. I had been fortunate to be able to use private insurance through Petro-Canada and even though I had left the company I was able to use a number of benefits until March 3rd, 2010. Doctor von Oertzen was happy with my progress and said that I could come off Clobazam. However, as I had experienced before, everything has withdrawal symptoms – although these where not as bad as before as the dosage was reduced very slowly. The worst part was the sleepless nights and being so tired. It was making me feel miserable and sorry for myself. The side-effects for most seizure tablets include drowsiness, dizziness, decreased appetite, shaking, confusion, unsteadiness, headaches, loss of memory and double vision. Sounds lovely, doesn't it?

The doctor said that as I would be on only one tablet after the 3rd March I could drive again, and I could have children if I wanted to as well, although not necessarily at the same time! I didn't want the children, but it was nice to know although I have found that it always helps to have a man first! It was great seeing the bars come down from my jail. It really had felt like a jail sometimes.

On Monday 1st March I woke up feeling very, very sick. This time it was not from feeling ill, just with butterflies as I was going to see Dr Minhas, my surgeon. It had been six months since I saw him last. All the way to the hospital I just wanted to throw up. It might seem silly but when you have all but lived in a hospital with all the appointments and the operations you can't help but develop a natural feeling of anticipation, fear and worry. I started to relax a little when thank God, Dr Minhas said he was happy with my MRI scan. However, even though he was pleased he said there was a tiny light part on the X-ray that might be more than it should be. He said he was not hugely worried, but he did say that although normally the next scan would be in a year, he would like me to have an X-ray in three months' time. That was a bit of a blow, and I knew I could not rest until I got a totally clear result. I had had good news, and most people would think I should be happy with that, but for me, only an all clear would put my mind totally at rest.

It was March 2010, and I was settled on the tablets, and the scan was positive, and I could relax slightly. Finally, I was ready for my trip to Thailand with Reka. We went to Bangkok, Phuket and Ko Samui. We knew it would be a great opportunity and I knew I needed to get out and about to feel more confident. I know most people would probably not take such a big step so early, but I have never done things by half. It was a very relaxing holiday, not too strenuous. We were up early and went to bed early. We were real partygoers – not! I saw the most amazing things. I was not always very forward with buying things or asking for help as my speech was not great and I was worse when I was panicking. I let Reka do that part as I didn't want to risk muddling my words up and any math's skills I might have had had gone right out of the window since the surgery. We returned home on the 18th, and it took me a whole week to get over it. The exhaustion was worth it though.

Once I had settled back in at home, a lady from Petro-Canada's insurance company came to meet me and said she would still help me get back to work again with a company that would understand and be sympathetic to my situation. It was nice that Petro-Canada wanted to help me even though I didn't work there anymore. After talking through my history, she said she would be in touch in about a month with some ideas for my future. I explained my recent visit to the hospital to her and the fact that the consultant thought there was a small chance that the tumour was still there, but I so wanted to go along with the idea I said I was sure it would be fine.

A month went by, and the lady from Petro-Canada came to see me a few times in May to sort out my going back to work. She would look through the options for jobs. If I am being honest, she was no help at all, sorry, but it is true. I could see that I was going to have to take charge of my life and not rely on others to give me the help I needed.

On Tuesday 4th of May, I had a phone call from the recruitment lady I had been dealing with in January. Although I had not been in a position to take the role in January, I was surprised and happy when she came up with a new role as a PA in a London Bridge company. I wasn't sure if I was going to be strong enough to take it yet. A busy PA role might be a little full-on seeing as how I was not a quick as I had been. I needed to think about it hard as I didn't want to make the wrong decision. Going for a job and then not being up to it would undoubtedly do me more harm than good. The lady I was dealing with, from Petro-Canada, said she thought it was a bad idea and I shouldn't go for the job. It was hard walking away from the opportunity as I had always worked, and not working felt like a failure. It made me feel like I wasn't good enough but, maybe this was something I was going to have to get used to.

The next month was all a bit of a blur. I was looking for work but was conscious that I wasn't going to settle on somewhere I would not be happy in. In July I had an eye test to see if they had improved and my peripheral vision was better. I was so nervous when I had it. I already knew when they gave me the results, they weren't good enough to drive again. I was hitting thing like tables and people all the time because I couldn't see them. I received a letter from the eye clinic who confirmed that I'd never drive again. It was hard. I felt so sick for days – I was shaking. One of my absolute joys was driving. I cried for days, and even to this day, I feel sick when I think that I will never get to drive again. I don't think I will ever be happy with not driving. I think it was the waiting that was hard. I still think about it when I really feel like just getting up and going on a road trip, but I have gotten used to using the train now, and it is not the end of the world. I just must ask a friend to drive if I want to go to somewhere, I can't get the train to.

Finally, on the 9th July 2010, I got a much more positive letter – the MRI scan showed that I was all clear. I did not need to be scared anymore. I would not need another X-ray for a year, such a relief.

At the end of July, Emma and George were getting married in Poland. I was nervous, as it was my first big event since before the tumour was removed. I was going to be a bridesmaid! My worst nightmare was being in front of people I didn't know (well some I did, obviously). I had about five panic attacks over the whole thing, but I was still determined to do it and felt very lucky to have been asked to be a bridesmaid and celebrate the special day. The wedding was in Poland as George is Polish, and they were getting married in beautiful Krakow. The whole trip and the wedding went well, and I had a few Coronas/glasses of wine to help with the nerves. I was glad once it was over but only because it was totally out of my comfort zone. The wedding was beautiful.

When I came home, I was trying to plan how to get back to work and have some sort of career plan again. Unfortunately, because it had taken so long to really get back on track again with work my confidence had feeling suffered? Finally, in September, I was asked by the job centre if I wanted to join another rehabilitation Centre called Attend ABI (Acquired Brain Injury). I immediately jumped at the opportunity, as I would take any help to get back to where I had been before all this. Attend ABI is a service that helps people with an acquired brain injury back to work. They provide training and support to help clients back into volunteering, education and the workplace. It shocked me, as they want nothing in return but want only to help. They are part of the 'Kings Fund'. Attend is designed for adults of working age who have an acquired non-progressive brain injury. If you have substantially completed your medical rehabilitation or need additional support to return to work, then Attend ABI can help you. The programme provides you with specialist neuro-rehabilitation services to help manage the cognitive, behavioural and emotional effects of brain injury. The programme includes specialist occupational assessment and planning services, and structured 'real world' work placements, as well as rehabilitative support both inside and outside of the workplace.

On the first day, I joined Attend ABI, the 1st of November 2010, I was feeling very positive but very nervous. They were based in London near Oxford Circus, in a beautiful building very near to Harley Street. I immediately liked the people I was learning with, and the staff. I was the only girl in a class of eight. I'd be lying if I said I didn't like all the attention. We were all around the same age but from totally different backgrounds.

The course lasted for three months. During December I went to spend Christmas with Emma and George in Dubai for a week and then flew over to Sydney to see Ian for New Year's Eve, courtesy of the tax rebate I had received. I wanted to push myself to get out and about on my own and build up my confidence which seemed to be an endless battle.

I had a lovely time. It was very relaxing, and I really appreciated the time away. Once I was back from my holidays, I went back to Attend ABI for a few more weeks. It was time to put everything I had learnt together and then start looking for work again.

I really had learnt a lot from Attend ABI. The things I discovered from there and from the other people on the course were so helpful and helped me a lot.
I learnt that it was OK to need a lot more rest than I was used to. I learnt not to beat myself up for being 'lazy'. Brain trauma from any cause leads to physical fatigue. It

takes a lot of energy, and it is very tiring for our brains to think, process, and organised.

I learnt that energy levels fluctuate and that even though we may look good or seem to be 'all better' on the outside, that might not be the case on the inside! Cognition is a fragile function for a brain tumour survivor. Some days are better than others. Pushing too hard usually leads to setbacks, sometimes even to illness.

Brain tumour recovery takes a very long time; it can take 10, 20 or more years. It continues long after formal rehabilitation has ended. And it can be exhausting trying to live up to the heartfelt desire of those around us who are expecting us to be back to exactly who we were, because, superficially, we look better.

We are not difficult if we resist social situations. Crowds, confusion, and loud sounds quickly overload our brains, which don't filter sounds as well as they used to.

Limiting our exposure is a coping strategy, not a behavioural problem!

If there is more than one person talking, we may seem to drift. That is because we have trouble following all the different threads of conversation. It is exhausting to keep trying to piece it all together. If you live with a brain injury patient or a brain tumour survivor, try to notice the circumstances if a behaviour problem arises. Our 'behaviour problems' are often an indication of an inability to cope with a specific situation. We may be frustrated, in pain, overtired or there may be too much confusion or noise for our brain to filter.

Please have patience with our memory. Keep in mind that not remembering does not mean that we don't care.

If we need to do tasks the same way all the time, it is because we are retraining our brain. It's like learning main roads before you can learn the shortcuts. Repeating tasks in the same sequence is a rehabilitation strategy.

If we seem sensitive, it could be a result of our brain tumour or its removal, and it may be a reflection of the extraordinary effort it takes to do things now. Tasks that used to feel automatic and take minimal effort now take much longer, require the implementation of numerous strategies and are huge accomplishments for us. Be patient with us! Don't confuse hope with denial. We are learning more and more about our amazing brains, and there are recorporalable stories about healing in the news every day. No-one can know for certain what our potential is. We need HOPE to be able to employ the many, many coping mechanisms, accommodations and strategies we need to navigate our new lives. Every single thing in our lives is extraordinarily difficult for us now. It would be easy to give up – without hope.

The Attend ABI course finished in February 2011. Through their support, I started to volunteer at St Christopher's Hospice in Sydenham. It was about 30 minutes from my house. I was there every day for around two months. It was strange at first being in a hospice. It was sad to think that the people there were often at the end of their lives. I was helping on the 'fundraising side'. I couldn't answer the phone, and they understood my fear of the telephone after a seizure back in 2009 was caused by a phone call. My role at the hospice was looking for businesses that could donate prizes for the various charity events they held. I loved working at the hospice. It gave me a purpose, and it felt good helping others.

Although everything was going well at the hospice, I knew I still needed to find a paid job. I got in touch with a recruitment agency and got a few interviews in London. It was not going well as I was getting interviews, but for one reason or another, the jobs offered were not appropriate for me anymore. My CV screamed 'Admin/PA' but that was not realistic, I just would not be able to do justice to that typically very busy role, I knew that. I went to some agencies to see if there was something a bit easier as I needed to ease my way back into work full time and not overdo it after this big gap in my CV.

Time to Ask for Help

The volunteering at St Christopher's Hospice was great I was working 7hr days but working every other day, so I could always rest in between. As it was in the fundraising office, it was not too demanding. After a few days, I found my sleep was beginning to be very restless again. At first, I thought it was because I was spending too much time thinking about my life and wanting to work – constantly wondering where I would go from here, where I would get a paid job and what kind of role I could realistically take on. I was getting further and further away from what I had been like before my operation, and I was looking for answers again. I was starting to find it hard to pray or even have an understanding of what I was going to do about my future. It is not a nice feeling when you have no goals, or at least when you can't even recognise a goal for yourself that you could realistically achieve.

I was having severe panic attacks in the day and even more at night. I think it was from my constant worry about life and what I would do. The attacks would always feel like the start of a seizure. They weren't, but it is hard not to have the fear of seizures in the back of your mind after you have had experience of them. And although I am not epileptic with flashing/strobe lights, I always felt as though I should not look at them as I felt they could easily trigger a seizure. It was suggested I should see a psychic to see if he or she could do a reading to make me feel at ease and to reassure me that everything would be OK with my future, but that was not a good idea for me. I have never given much thought to that kind of thing and never really wanted to get involved or entertain the subject, as it is not something, I believe in. It is strange how you will go to a great extent to find answers.

I was given a number for a popular psychic and even though every part of my body said, "Don't do it", I did. Maybe it was me rebelling against my own faith as things were going wrong again and I was getting depressed with all the ups and downs of my recovery.

So, I spoke to the psychic. She said all good things and told me that everything would be fine and gave me some more information. What she said was enlightening, but after I had the reading, my nightmares and paranoia got worse and worse. I was constantly feeling there was something in the room with me. The lady I spoke to said it was my spiritual guides and they were there to help me with my decisions. That really freaked me out.

For weeks after I was afraid of the strange feeling, I had like something was always there. I wished the lady didn't say I had a spiritual guide with me always. I prayed for forgiveness, and I asked my Christian friends to pray with me over the situation. Soon the bad feeling had gone, but I was still struggling with where I should go from here.

Roland had told me to look up a particular sermon by Pastor Jesse Duplantis, who is one of my favourite pastors from America. The sermon was about how much God loves us and what he has waiting for us one day and how he wouldn't let anything happen to me as I am his child. I felt better already.

I sent Jesse Duplantis an email to pray for me and explained my situation. A lady called me from his ministry, and then she prayed for me on the phone. Two days later I was given the opportunity to interview for my friend Amanda's company. I thought "Wow that was quick, thank you, God." I got a second interview, and I got the job! I started the next week on the 28th of March, the day after my 28th birthday.

The job went well for the first few weeks, and I was getting on with everyone at work. I loved being back in the city. Getting up early and just being back to how I wanted to be, struggling into work along with all the other commuters, full of purpose for the day ahead. I knew the job was not easy but the fact I had Amanda there gave me a boost to try, and I was able to speak to her if I got stuck with anything. Can you believe I even met a guy at the company, and we went on a few dates? The relationship wasn't going anywhere, but at least I could see I was still in the game and had my swag! LOL.

Into the fourth week of my new job, I realised I was working nine-hour days, and that is not including the travel time there and back. So, I was actually doing eleven hours a day. I liked being busy, but my body was struggling; I was coming home and going straight to bed and then getting up for work. Now Amanda was getting married in April, and I was excited, as I was to be one of her bridesmaids. I knew this was going to be another trial, as I would have a very long and busy weekend and then must get straight back to work.

The wedding was terrific, and we had a lovely time. Amanda looked stunning. The night before the wedding Amanda, to observe tradition and not see her groom, had slept in my room. She said she noticed I was shaking in the night – my feet and legs were shaking. I had heard that people do have seizures at night and that this kind of shaking was a sign.

Monday came around all too soon, and it was time for work. I was so exhausted I couldn't even remember my name or what to say on the phone. I was forgetting messages. I was not with it at all. I felt like I was in a bubble that I needed to pop to get back out into the world around me.

It was April, and on the Thursday of that week we were all looking forward to the long weekend – the big royal wedding for Prince William and Kate. All the UK had a four-day holiday. I needed it badly to get back some energy. When I went back to work, I spoke to my supervisor. We talked about the situation, and we agreed it was not working. I should have been devastated, but I was glad. I had tried, and the experience had made me realise that no matter how much I wanted my life back to how it was, what I was trying to do was not realistic at all.

I went back to the hospice on Tuesday. I was tired, but I was doing OK, and then a week later I got flu again – go figure. I am a walking advert for lemon and honey! I knew I had really overdone it with the job in London and should have had a rest before I went to the hospice, but I just wanted to keep busy, so I did not get too comfortable being idle...

I really loved working at the hospice; we were setting up for another fun run. The day after the fun run we had to pick up all the water bottles that were left over. They were being looked after in Waitrose as it was close to where the fun run had been held.

There were only three of us, and there were hundreds of boxes with eight bottles in each. I have never claimed to be a manual person. I can just about lift my head these days let alone lift boxes. After having got all the boxes on the van we went to drive off and bang, the tyre blew. I laughed, it shows how heavy the cargo was. We waited around for three-quarters of an hour until the AA turned up to change the tyre. Back at the hospice, we had to take all the boxes back off the van and put them onto some trolleys. I was fine doing stuff but knew this wasn't the great thing for me to do with so little energy.

I finally got home and went straight to bed. It was one of those moments when you hit the pillow you are out like a light. I woke up about 09:00 and was feeling very tired – my body was aching. I went to go and wash my face and locked the door. I knew Mum was just outside the door. Next thing I knew I was back on the floor wondering "Did I have a seizure, or did I faint?" I was OK and was sure I had just fainted, nothing more. I just went back to bed and slept it off. I relaxed the whole day and then had an early night. I woke up early the next day at 05:30 as Mum and Dad were picking Ian and Phoebe up from the airport. They had had a long flight from Sydney, and I knew we needed to keep them up for the day. I did get up at 05:00 to say bye to my parents and was trying to stay awake but I was still fatigued from the bottle carrying. I said hello to Ian and Phoebe and told them I would have to just get some more sleep and then I would be more awake later.

I finally woke up and had a catch-up with them. It was so nice to see them. In the afternoon we went shopping in town and bought a game for my Wii. It was another guitar (Wii guitar). We went home and played on the games. It was good, but later that day I started really feeling my shoulder aching terribly. I realised it was the side I had fallen on. It was depressing at times when I wanted nothing more than to keep up with Ian and Phoebe while they were with us, and instead I had to keep resting. While Ian was home, we celebrated his 30th birthday. We had a huge family party for him. I had to keep taking rests in the day and went for a nap every now and then as I found it very loud with everyone in the house.

After the party I was pretty much bed bound relaxing, my shoulder was getting worse. While I was home, I had to do something to stop myself from going mad from boredom and worrying about myself. I hadn't really talked about my actual experience with other people very much. I had always kept this to myself, and I had never investigated what a brain tumour really was. It had been three years, but it was such a scary subject to me that I adopted a sort of head in the sand attitude.

But I felt a lot stronger in my mind now, and I finally wanted an understanding of brain tumours. I started looking at websites. I knew my situation but had never actually spoken to other brain tumour survivors or sufferers. I had met people at the Attend ABI, but they were all people who had had head injuries rather than brain tumours.

After looking at the various websites that were out there, I realised there were also forums on Facebook. I went to an American one first for meningioma patients. As I started reading the comments people were writing I began to cry. It was very hard reading about people's experiences and their struggles. It was nice to see the problems I was having were very normal. 'Normal', what on earth does that word mean?

I could see how hard people were finding their situations and I wanted to help. I think it also took my attention away from myself and tempered much of my introspection, which was a good thing. Somehow, I did not want my family and friends to hear me talking about my brain tumour journey and recovery because, as ridiculous as it sounds, I think I was embarrassed. It was as though it was my fault or that I was an embarrassment, with a disability. That seems so silly now, but I didn't meet anyone else in my position for three years after my surgery. After a few days of looking through the websites and forums on Facebook, I decided I wished there was a more positive website that really focused on cheering people up.

It was May 20th in 2011 and the anniversary of the day I had been to the optician three years earlier to find out that my eyes were bleeding at the back. It felt like a good day to start a new chapter in my life.

I set up a page on Facebook, and I called it 'Aunty Meningioma'. I did not want to give my name away at that point as I didn't want everyone to know who I was and didn't want my friends or family to see my true feelings about the whole thing. I also wanted to speak with others and didn't want my age to put people off. It was easier to make up a name, and I thought people might find the name 'Aunty' comforting.

Every morning, afternoon and evening I would put an encouraging but funny photo on the page to make people smile. Day by day more people were adding themselves to the page. People seemed to be really benefiting from my positive comments, and they were always related to brain tumours. It felt good.

Ian and Phoebe were still over, and every time somebody added to my Facebook page, I would say out loud '1 more yay'. I think they all thought I was being a little strange and people wanted me to move on, but in my mind, this was just the beginning of my recovery and finally meeting others. Better late than never I say. Ian and Phoebe returned to Sydney after their three-week holiday with us. It was sad seeing them go, but I was so glad they came to see us.

Once they had gone back to Sydney, I was still having trouble with my shoulder. It was very painful. One night it got so bad I almost went to casualty to get some help. It was only through the fear that I would not be able to cope with the noise and confusion in casualty on a Saturday night that I decided to just put up with the pain and wait until Monday to go to the doctor.

I went back to see the doctor and mentioned that my neck was hurting from falling the week before and it wasn't getting better it was getting worse, and I was having terrible spasms. I thought it would be a good idea to mention that Amanda had noticed me shaking in the

night when I stayed over on her wedding night. The
doctor gave me some cream to help with my shoulder,
and he said I should ask somebody to sleep in the bed
with me and see if I did it again – so, with no takers on
being my bed buddy of the male variety, I asked my
mum to sleep with me! She did it for three nights, and
on each of the three nights, I did the same thing,
shaking. The GP doctor said I should speak to my seizure
doctor, Dr von Oertzen. He was away on holiday so while
I was waiting on Doctor von Oertzen, I decided to send
him an email to voice my concerns.

Dear Doctor, von Oertzen,
I know I have an appointment on the 27th June 2011,
but I am concerned. I have been having many problems
again with a lack of sleep and feeling very, very tired all
day. I am used to the tiredness, but now it has gotten
worse. I have been struggling with my speech again,
with finding words and with focusing. I find any kind of
noise is hard on my nerves; this has been going on for a
month. I have also been getting very tense in my
shoulders and feeling very sick, dizzy and disorientated. I
was not like this for a good two years, but it is very

unsettling. This was happening before I reduced my Tegretol Retard from 1000mg to 800mg. I thought the reduction would help but it is just stayed the same, and I am feeling very sick and nervous like I may have a seizure because of the tiredness and stress. Please help?

I have spoken to my GP already, and as usual, they just did a blood test which was for anemia and Tegretol levels which were normal, but I know my own body, and something is wrong. I never make a fuss normally, but I am nervous, and it is not nice to have been feeling sick and weak for nearly a month.
I look forward to hearing from you.
Claire

After my email, Dr von Oertzen set up a meeting for me with him. We met at St George's with other people observing us. I was feeling very low and had to really push myself, but I wanted some help, and how would they know what I needed if I couldn't speak up? Doctor von Oertzen said he wanted to wait for my MRI results to come through as I was due to have a scan any day –

that way he could dismiss the possibility that the problems I was having were tumour related.

I had the MRI a few weeks later and had an anxious wait for the results. It then took three weeks to hear the results as the hospital had misplaced my file. Once I met Dr Minhas again, he said he was sorry for the wait – I should never have had to wait so long to hear the results of my MRI. But it was all good news, and the MRI was fine. It was so nice to see a clear picture.

Dr Minhas said my problems may be arising from seizures. He thought we should set up an electroencephalogram (EEG). He said he would speak to Dr von Oertzen and discuss the next course of action.

A week later I got an official letter that said my scan was all clear and that there were no more problems from the surgical side. It went on to say that I might have depression. I was really hurt by this because when I had met Dr Minhas the previous week, we had agreed it was not depression and that the small seizures might be making me feel sick and very tired. I felt sad all weekend because I couldn't understand why he was now saying that my problems were due to depression. Maybe he was right, and I was just going mad.

Finally, I had a letter from the hospital again about the discussion with Dr Minhas. They said the letter was wrong and that it shouldn't have said I had depression. It was a copy of the one they had sent me six months earlier, but it was mislaid, so they sent it so I could have it in my files!

It did say they wanted to look into my seizure medication and that they would like me to have a few tests for my cognitive abilities. I then went to have some tests, and the results showed I definitely needed some cognitive therapy. They also set me up another appointment to see Dr von Oertzen, but he was on holiday, so I saw another seizure doctor. She was a lady I had never met before. She said from my symptoms that my problems were due to my seizures. She said I should go from 800mg Tegretol to 1600mg in a gradually increasing dose. They would set me up with a psychologist and a cognitive therapist.

While I was happy, we had a result I was sad that it was going to take time to stop experiencing that feeling in my body that a seizure was imminent. She told me to start a diary to track how I was feeling, to see when the seizures were occurring. I wrote the diary, and it seemed every night I was struggling with tension and funny feeling of falling,

Waiting for the tablets to kick in again took time. It took 10 weeks to get on the correct dosage, and I was still having very strange sensations and was waking up in the night shaking. I knew I had to hang in there, I knew it would start to get better soon.

I had got to 1400mg, and it was not working, and my seizures continued day and night, so it was not a great existence. I was waiting to see a shrink so I could talk about my problems as I was not leaving the house for fear I might end up jumping around in the street. I was becoming a recluse.

I didn't go out for over six months while the tablet dosage was still going up. I felt so unwell and tired it was absolutely exhausting.

On Friday 19th of October, I had a meeting with Doctor von Oertzen who was not happy with the previous doctor's course of action four to five months earlier. He said I had been put on the wrong tablets and I was not having seizures, it was just vivid dreams! Which would have set-off anxiety issues.

I spent from October to December adjusting to new tablets called Lamictal (Lamotrigine). Slowly! I was having endless problems with feeling sick, headaches, sickness, vision and low weight (the latter not necessarily a bad thing!).

I carried on with my Facebook page while I was stuck home. Still, I really learnt a lot from the people who shared their brain tumour experiences, and although they were seeing my pictures and posts, they would explain what their connection to a brain tumour was. At that point, I did not know enough about brain tumours to realise there are 120 types of brain tumour out there and that they are graded.

I had nearly 600 people on the page by September and realised maybe I should change the name as I didn't want to make it just for 'meningioma sufferers/survivors. I met Keith Davies, a fellow brain tumour patient who had a tumour called a parasagittal atypical meningioma. He was a similar age to me, and after sharing our brain tumour experiences he was very helpful, and we came up with the name Aunty M Brain Tumours. We devised a catchy introduction to tell people what I did and to make them feel very welcome.

Wall:
"Join Aunty M who is all about positive thinking and is a place to meet friends who understand about brain tumours. The thing we all seek in life is to get through the hard times and keep smiling. I was diagnosed with an Intraventricular meningioma in 2008. I have been through it and still am going through it, but I am on my way out the other side now, and I am staying positive!

Eventually, in December, I ventured out and turned the laptop off. I was so paranoid that I might have a seizure. Although I had finished the swap-over with the tablets, I was still having trouble with anxiety and worry. Unfortunately, the one time I did go out to do some Christmas shopping I caught a cold – typical.

I went to meet Dr von Oertzen again to reassess my situation and what we could do, going forward. I was feeling nervous as I had been hiding in the safe cocoon of my home. Dr von Oertzen was happy that I was going to get counselling and said we would see how I got on with that.

When I left the appointment, I was not feeling very confident as I was told I would be on seizure tablets my whole life. He said my hippocampus had been damaged in the surgery and there was a lot of scarring that would trigger seizures. Being me and being in central London, Mum and I went to a few shops to browse and try to regain our equilibrium after the rather depressing news. I bought some nice things and managed to forget about the meeting for a short while. Back on the train and back to West Norwood, we got the bus up the hill. I was listening to my iPod, and then it hit me. Damn! I won't ever get off the meds! I glanced over and saw a person reading a newspaper. On the back, it said in big letters 'SHAME'. That was just what I wanted to see! It would have been funny if it were not so tragic!

I got home and felt bad for a few minutes and then squared my shoulders and decided I would just have to get on with it.

Doctor von Oertzen reiterated to my GP that I needed to go and do some cognitive counselling and some counselling specifically for people who have had brain surgery. I was feeling positive about that. I didn't sleep all night. I started watching some TV and then suddenly on the news they were talking about 'cognitive behaviour'. They were explaining everything, and I was just thinking "Thank you, Lord, good timing."

I understood now it was not about being slow or just strange. Cognitive problems were like a person who has had their mind set put into the wrong video machine. All I needed to do was to get the right one back to carry on!

It is not a quick process. It takes a long time but with determination, I know I will get there.

I spent Christmas on my own. I was meant to go to my uncle's house for Christmas Day, but my cousin had just been diagnosed with Hodgkin's Lymphoma, so it was not a good idea to spread my germs to him. I was more than happy on the sofa with a lot of feel good movies and my lemon and honey drinks. Thank goodness for 'Sky Movies'!

Finally, I got to talk to my GP and got her talking with my seizure doctor's assistant, as Dr von Oertzen was away on holiday. I think they felt sorry for me as it was Christmas, so they tried to sort me out, which I really appreciated.

They said there must be some other reason for my symptoms. I spent the night feeling so unlucky, only to be reassured the next day that all my symptoms were not from my seizures. I was having panic attacks and anxiety attacks. I then had to speak to my GP and set up a meeting with a counsellor. As it was Christmas, I had to wait until after the New Year celebrations.

After working tirelessly on Aunty M Brain Tumours through Christmas, I decided the blog etc. was working well, and within 15 months I had over 13,000 people connecting on my different websites.

On December 31st I was going to spend New Year's Eve with me, myself and I, but I was glad I had a plan. Ding Dong! It was January 1st, 2012. Can you believe it? I slept through it as I was fast asleep by 22:00 lol. It was nice to speak with brain tumour warriors around the world on the 'Aunty M's Facebook page. It was not such a lonely Christmas as there were others in the same situation and we were all there together to say goodbye to the year and bring on the new one.

Starting from Scratch

Once all the Christmas holidays were over, and the decorations were back in the loft, it was time to make some New Year resolutions. I had a new diary to share my journey. Although my working life had ended, for now, I was determined to turn Aunty M Brain Tumours into something more for me and or other people like me.

Now I found myself again in a round of hospital appointments. I got a letter from the Neurologist who had been dealing with my seizures for the past four years. The letter explained that he thought that I would benefit from seeing a CBT practitioner. It was something I had discussed with him before Christmas because I was struggling with anxiety prompted by my fear of having seizures.

What the heck is CBT I thought? I immediately went to investigate on Google.

"Cognitive Behavioral Therapy (CBT) encompasses some practical and helpful strategies that can be incorporated into everyday life, and that will help a person cope better with future stresses and difficulties even after the treatment has finished. CBT involves confronting your emotions and anxieties; CBT only addresses current problems and focuses on specific issues and how to cope with them".

Well, it sounded interesting, and I always say I'll try anything once!

As I was going through the NHS, I was on a waiting list, and my first CBT session wouldn't be until November. The NHS has many good things, but the downside is the waiting time for any appointments for therapy. My GP said that while I was waiting, I could see a standard counsellor to just talk about how I felt about everything. I never say no to some 'Counselling' you never know, one day it might, surprisingly, work.

I was starting to feel very 'Sex and The City'. I remembered the quote by Carrie Bradshaw 'First they want you to come there two times a week, then three times a week, and eventually you're starting every sentence with 'my therapist says'.

In my appointments, the counsellor listened to me talking about my fears about having seizures. I told him my experiences and how they scared me so much. I explained it felt it was ingrained in my mind, right up there with the fact if I go in any room where I should lock the door, like a bathroom, I always keep my phone with me, or the door is open. All because I had a grand-mal seizure behind a locked closed door and could not get out. That terrifying incident had taken a significant toll on my confidence. I explained that it seemed the more tired I was, the more anxious I would feel when I was in noisy places. I'd have a terrible feeling that at any moment I might have a seizure. That very thing had unfortunately happened a few times three years earlier, and I had never got over the terrifying experience.

After a few sessions with my local doctor's counsellor, I had an appointment at St George's hospital for a check-up at the neuropsychiatry clinic. The doctor highlighted the fact that although I was feeling slightly more confident, I was still not sure enough to go out alone. He said that it was very common for people suffering from seizures to develop panic attacks and avoidance behaviour.

He was right; when I went out, I would always have to have somebody with me, I hadn't even realised that I was doing that. The psychiatrist gave me anxiety tablets and said that with the medication and the CBT sessions that I would be having in November, should improve things even more.

Spring came, and now I was celebrating the 4th year since I had my craniotomy (brain surgery), or as the brain tumour community call it, a Cranniversary. I had to admit that the time since those first terrifying days had flown by, even if it did not always feel like it. I felt fortunate I have survived the experience. I know my life had been changed forever and things are nowhere near the life I would have liked. But I was determined not to wallow in my very own pity party, and I knew that I needed a project to work on.

Then I got an unexpected lifeline, my Godmother told me she was going abroad over the summer to spend a few weeks in Turkey and invited me to join her if I wanted to. I decided to see it as a 'Cranniversary' gift to myself and was grateful to be asked. I booked my trip and flew out a week later. I took my laptop, and I planned to sit by the pool finishing my first book 'A Brain Tumour's Travel Tale'.

What I was determined to do was turn the diaries and journals I had kept, detailing what had happened to me into a book that wasn't just for my family but that other people could read and hopefully find some hope or inspiration from the book.

But part of my condition was that I was often a bit forgetful, and I left the laptop charger at home! With only 4hrs left on the battery, I was limited to how much time I could work on the book. The result was that I had the rest of the 11days by the pool relaxing and reading magazines. Not the worst accident to have but it did mean that I would have to make up the time when I got back.

After my holiday, I finished my book. I started a search for someone online who could check my grammar and knock my writing into shape. I came across a lady called Amanda T. I went to meet her, and I told her what I wanted. She was very sympathetic to what I had been through and said to me that, it would take her about three weeks to get it done. I was so proud of myself. I was really making this thing happen now!

While I was waiting for Amanda to send me her transcript, I was looking for ways to keep my costs down for publishing the book and learnt how to self-publish a Kindle eBook via YouTube. It was not as easy a process as you might think. I'm a slow learner now, but I always get there eventually. I never give up once I have my mind set on something!

Summer came and with it some great news. St George's Hospital called me to say my MRI scans would now be undertaken every two years instead of each year. That was wonderful; I was looking forward to moving away from that episode in my life and felt confident that it was behind me now.

Eventually, after finding my way through the complicated machinations of self-publishing, my book was finally ready to go live on Kindle. To keep my costs down, I had learned how to jump through the hoops necessary with the help of YouTube. While this was happening, my friend said she would tell the local newspaper about my eBook and see if they would cover it. Within a week I was contacted by the Croydon Advertiser who stated that they wanted to cover the story and would send a photographer to take some photos of me with the book! It was a great result.

Then, my interview was there for everyone to see, in the newspaper! I woke up at 5 am, with butterflies in my tummy. I drank a few mugs of hazelnut coffee to give me the boost I needed to walk around to my local newsagent so early. With trembling fingers, I opened the paper and there I was! Right there on the inside page were my photo and my story giving details about the new book. I was thrilled; the man who had written the article had done a great job. It was so exciting!

Within a week of the article, a PR lady called Kirsty, contacted me. Kirsty wanted to cover my story and my brain tumour experience for a piece for Bella Magazine. This was something I had not expected, and I was very flattered. I did, however, worry that if I did share my story with this National audience, I was basically announcing to any prospective employer out there that I was unemployable. More than anything I did want to be able to earn money again and be independent again one day.

On the other hand, there was the fact that sharing my experience might help others who were in the early stages of their brain tumour journey. I had to be less concerned about myself and concentrate more on the fact that I was now becoming an advocate and a voice for the brain tumour community. So, I said yes. She came over to go through my story and told me that the article would be published in December, in the Christmas special edition.

Continuing what felt like a lucky streak, I decided I would consider other ways to promote my book. I was Googling 'How To...' pages and where to go to get exposure. On one suggested that a good way to get publicity was to get on local radio stations. At first, I thought 'No Way'! The prospect of speaking on the radio seemed just too scary. A week later, I thought I would look into the radio option again. I had had a week to calm my initial nerves at the thought of it and to talk myself into it. I saw there was a new local online radio station in Croydon. I sent an email to ask if they would be interested in my coming in to talk about my book. Two weeks later I had an email back from one of their radio presenters, Maria Kay. She said they would be keen to interview me before the end of the year. We agreed that I would go into the radio station on the 20th December.

I asked my Mum to come along with me for moral support. When I was about to go in the studio, I did suffer a bit of stage fright or maybe more accurately, 'vocal fright' as obviously, being radio, nobody can see you. I asked Mum if she could come into the actual recording booth with me. Her face registered a look of surprise as I pulled my most needy face to plead with her to go in. To my surprise, she did agree. We talked about the book, and Maria asked Mum and me about our experience, about my recovery and the on-going medical problems I have had. Where I was nervous about speaking up Mum couldn't stop talking. Overall the interview went great, and after the show, we went to get a coffee with Maria just to say thanks. While we were sipping our drinks, Maria said I had a good voice for radio and if I wanted, I could do a trial day for a slot at the station. Well, you could have knocked me over with a feather! Me? On the radio?

I realised the radio had only been running for 11 months, and that they were still expanding trying to introduce a broad range of programs, some music and some talk shows. Volunteers ran it all. Maria said all I had to do was come up with a show name and what I wanted to talk about and then apply for the role online.

I said I would have to go and have a think about it and come back to her. I was stunned. I wrote a post on my website and the Facebook Page, to try and gauge what people would want to hear. I wanted them to find whatever I did choose as a theme, to be beneficial. While I was waiting for feedback at the end of December, my story appeared in Bella Magazine. It was an excellent piece, but I was starting to realise that magazines will always slightly spin the story you give them to meet their own agenda. But I was happy that it was still raising awareness for brain tumours, and that was my ultimate goal.

Brain Tumour Thursday Radio Show

At the beginning of January, it was eye-check time, or should I say reality check time? I went to St George's for the assessment of my peripheral vision. Unfortunately, that had not improved, and I had to face the fact that the eyesight I had was what I was going to have to live with now, forever. With a New Year dawning, it was a bit of a blow to start that year off. On the plus side, my eyes hadn't got worse, so I would just carry on and keep waiting for my visual miracle. And I knew that I could wait! I had waited this long, I was determined that I was not going to get disheartened. I just waited patiently for God to guide me and keep me positive no matter what I was faced with.

I was finally seeing a new cognitive behavioural therapist. I was to have 12 sessions, and I was optimistic that I would see a difference in my mindset and confidence with my disabilities. It is unusual to have a handsome man who was pleasant to the eye as a therapist. I found it slightly intimidating. I struggled initially to feel comfortable and to speak openly. He gave me some great examples of what anxiety was. What I understood was that anxiety was the body building up to some event like an adrenaline rush before a race. The problem was that I was not running a race, so in me that energy had nowhere to go and the result was that I would freak out.

I also had to talk about presumptions. I had an idea that as far as other people were concerned my brain tumour and my recovery were well behind me, and I was now back to full health. Unfortunately, that was not the case. I was living with on-going disabilities, that were invisible to others, and it was hard to believe people wanted to hear what was happening. Over the 12 weeks, I did see a difference in the way I looked at things. It was helpful as it put my life in perspective and I recognised that I had come a very long way from my surgery.

All this did not stop me worrying about seizures, however, but what it did do was help with helping me to understand what panic actually feels like. I needed to acknowledge that I hadn't had a seizure for a very long time and to trust that my seizure medication was working. In turn, I needed to trust my body and remind myself that the feelings that came over me were panic, not the onset of a seizure.

Now I will try to talk myself out of the anxiety feeling. I do feel scared, but then I can say to myself "It is just an adrenaline rush, it will pass, everything is going to be ok, relax Claire".

I put more thought into the possibility of being a presenter on Croydon Radio. In my heart, I felt that it was a great opportunity and as it was volunteering, it would be less stressful than paid work. I did question myself though, would I be able to deal with my anxiety or fumbling words. I decided I needed to woman-up and went to the station for the trial day.

I arrived at Matthews Yard in Croydon, which is where the station was based. I had no idea what this interview would involve or what would happen there, just that I would share my idea and my possible radio show name for them to consider. My Mum came with me, for moral support. She was going to wait in the coffee shop. I was so nervous, and when I got talking about my show idea, I said I was going to do a mother and daughter duo. Mum could talk about being the carer of someone who has had a brain tumour, and I could share my knowledge from the patient's point of view. The idea was that I would connect with people through my social media platforms. I would call it "The Brain Tumour Thursday Show" as it tied in with the universal online campaign 'Brain Tumour Thursday'. We would play uplifting music, invite people to tell their stories and interview representatives of the various brain tumour charities as well as experts from the medical field. I had no idea if it would work or if Mum would even agree to do it with me. To my surprise, she said yes and went along with what I was saying. My Mum is so supportive, and I know how fortunate I am to have such a great relationship with her.

The Radio managers said we were welcome to join the team. And we would start with our first show on the 31st of January. We were excited. We would be doing 2hr shows. I spent hours looking online finding ways in which I could help to make my show easy to listen too. I put together an introduction for listeners to hear:

"Aunty M & Eileen B, time to make a cup of tea. We are here to brighten up your lunchtime with great music and positive messages to any person affected by a brain tumour; but more than that, we are here to encourage anyone who needs a boost on a Thursday afternoon. Every Thursday people around the world share facts, statistics and stories all day long in the hope of spreading awareness of brain tumours. I myself 'Aunty M' am a brain tumour survivor, so I know how important it is to keep active and encouraged. Grab a cuppa and sit back while Eileen B and myself entertain you with our uplifting show! We will play a range of music and would love to hear from you on the Shoutbox, tell us how your day is going. We are here for sufferers, survivors, family, friend or anyone needing a pick-me-up".

I prepared my first show and asked people:

"If you have had an MRI scan before, you will know that it sounds like you have been plonked down in the middle of a construction site. If you were going to make a playlist to hear on a CD in the MRI scan, what would be your picks?"

I said once suggestions were sent in, I would play the chosen song during the show and give a shout-out to whoever had sent in the suggestion.

A great bonus was that although the shows were going to be live, they were also put onto a podcast which meant that people in Europe, America, Australia, or further afield could hear us whenever they wanted to.

When the 31st came, and we made our debut, you could hear how nervous we were. I was struggling to find words, and I'd be waving my arms around and pulling faces to get Mum's attention. She would then just jump in because she knew what I was trying to say. Thank goodness nobody could see us looking like deer in the headlights. I knew that I wouldn't have coped without her.

As we said our goodbyes to the listeners, put our last song on and went to the crossover with the next presenter, I realised we hadn't put the podcast on so that show was never to be heard again. Oops, it was certainly a learning curve it was a good thing as we had now had our warm-up show and would be ready for a more polished performance the following week.

I was exhausted after the first day. As soon as I got home, I went straight to bed for a nap. But I had enjoyed the experience so much that I could not wait to research my next show that would be aired, the following week.

I asked people on my social networking sites for any methods they had used to combat the times that they were feeling fatigued. Everything was all set for the following week, and we even remembered to put the podcast on, phew!

In February, the show was building up a great following, and we could see from the stats that lots of people were tuning in to the live show and even more on the podcast. It wasn't just people in the UK; people were listening all around the world. All this was doing wonders for my confidence and mum loved her new celebrity status as 'Eileen B' in charge of the music side of things!

My recruitment skills from my working days were really helping me with interviewing guests. I have always loved watching how Piers Morgan puts people at ease on 'Piers Morgan's Life Stories'. He is brilliant at it, and I tried to emulate him in my technique.

Back to reality and I was again at the hospital for a check-up with my neuropsychiatrist. I told him that the cognitive behavioural therapy had helped me, but that I was still concerned about my lack of sleep and how I found certain noises intolerable which in turn seemed to heighten my anxiety even though I was on medication. He gave me sleeping tablets and said they should help. He would also send my GP a form to set me up to see a hearing specialist to see if there was a problem with my hearing that might be causing some of the issues. I walked out with my cocktail of pills and prescriptions, and I was feeling confident that at last the concerns I had were being looked into. I was also pleased that I had remembered everything that I wanted to ask.

I worked hard on promoting the radio show and getting as many guests as I could to share their experiences or to talk about the charities they supported. In doing that, I had some fantastic opportunities to share my story. I wanted to raise as much awareness as possible. I was learning so much on my own journey now and from my interviews with others.

In March, I gave my first ever talk. It was at Friends of O.S.C.A.R. Friends of O.S.C.A.R is a support group in Oxfordshire; a charity set up to help children with brain and spinal tumours and their families throughout the country. I was very nervous, but I put on my game face and shared my story. As I looked around the hall, it was mainly parents who had a child dealing with a brain tumour. They were, of course, desperately concerned for their child, and I pray I gave them hope that life can go on when you have a brain tumour, and I hope that I also provided them with some comfort that we as patients are all so much stronger than we realise.

I was also interviewed by a radio show to share my story as part of International Women's Day. I was enjoying myself, but I was still suffering from terrible panic attacks. I refused to let them stop me doing things, but boy they were horrible. The noisier the place, the more my heart rate would go up. The more my heart rate went up, the more confused I would feel. I would just be looking for the right word. I'd ask God to calm me. It amazes me how people never could tell what a fight I was having in my mind, I was so grateful for that. People said I should make a book called 'Claireis-amz'. Maybe one day I will, but let's get this one out the way first!

By July, Mum and I had graduated to meeting people attending for their hospital appointments who were willing to share their experiences with my listeners. Some people would be having radiotherapy or chemotherapy. Everyone was going through a terrible time, but they were all managing, in their own way.

One of my Facebook Page fans, called Lily asked if I could help promote a film called 'These Three Words'. It was a documentary feature about five individuals facing brain cancer, finding hope, love and life. Lily explained that the director of the movie, the main star of the film and their Assistant Theresa were travelling to England from Rhode Island to meet the scientist who had been responsible for producing a chemo drug called Temozolomide (Temedol), which all five were currently taking.

The scientists were in Birmingham, and the team would be in London on their trip, and they asked if they could be interviewed on my radio show. I said yes, of course.

The Americans

In August, England was in the middle of a heat wave, and the temperatures were sizzling in the 30's. I told all my radio listeners I was going to have The 'These Three Words' team on the show the following week and made the joke that I would maybe get the hip-hop artist's phone number if he were single. Obviously, this was tongue in cheek.

I had set up a day for the producer Paul and the star of the film Andrew Reis (Ace Diamond) to be interviewed on the 8th and Andrew would talk about the film, and as they were only in London for three days, I offered to put all three of them up at my house.

On the 7th August, they arrived and understandably, were still a little jet-lagged. They enthralled us by telling us all about the film and all the things they had been shooting over the last four years.

After a lovely meal that my mother cooked, I decided I
needed to take a break. The room was getting noisy with
all the different animated conversations. As usual, I
could only cope with one sound at a time. I asked
Andrew to sing something for me. His face was a picture.
"What! Right now?" I laughed and said

"No, come upstairs, we can get my equipment out I
already have a ready-made studio from being a karaoke
junkie in my college days. I explained I used to set up
karaoke nights when I was in college to earn a bit of
money." Sure". He said.

I started singing first and hoped that he didn't put his
fingers in his ears, but he seemed quite impressed with
my vocals. I happened to have the backing track for
Rhianna with 'Diamonds' in the disc player. I know, I
know, very corny, I sang it anyway!

Once I'd warmed up the room, and done my bit, I
handed over the microphone to Andrew. I was excited
as I had heard him rapping online, but I hadn't heard him
sing in any other genre. When he started, I all but

melted. He had such a soulful voice, very sexy. I could hear echoes of Marvin Gaye in my mind humming 'Let's Get It On'.

Once we had done our solo performances, we got the duets out. It was so much fun, I could have sung with him all night, and I could see he was having as much fun as I was.

Once we had exercised our vocal cords, I suggested hot chocolate drinks with marshmallows. I like to think of myself as a hot chocolate connoisseur, so I was in my comfort zone.

Andrew was so easy to talk to. We chatted for hours and continued to share our experiences and talk about our childhoods. We talked about music, about our faith and our hopes and dreams for the future. It was much later before we realised everyone was fast asleep in the house, and we really should get some rest. As Andrew was leaving my room, we could hear Paul snoring like a foghorn. Andrew was not impressed, as he was going to be sleeping in the same room as Paul. We looked at each other and laughed. I made a joke saying, 'You can stay in my room on the floor if you like'. I didn't think for a second that he would take up my offer. I was a bit embarrassed to have said anything really because I wasn't sure where he was going to sleep.

As it was a boiling hot night, and nobody needed to sleep under a duvet just a sheet, I put my duvet on the floor to make it less uncomfortable and provide some sort of a mattress for Andrew as well as some pillows to sleep on.

I asked if he was sure it was comfortable enough. He said he didn't have a bed at home, and he was used to sleeping on the floor. I was thinking, 'Thank goodness for that' when he started laughing, and I realised that he was pulling my leg. I just raised my eyebrow and smiled back.

I did have every intention of sleeping; I was exhausted, and I really was struggling to keep my eyes open. Andrew was still wide awake at 2 am; I guessed that was because he was in Rhode Island time which was 5hrs behind the UK and we carried on talking although I was mumbling most of my words, I was so tired I kept drifting in and out of sleep and in and out of the conversation. It was so effortless to speak with Andrew, it really was like talking to a best friend. We talked about everything, and I was astonished to find myself sharing with him, things I wouldn't usually share with people, and I think he felt the same.

We discovered that both of us wanted to set up our own foundations where people who had been affected by a brain tumour could go for support and because we were both such huge music fanatics, we would do a charity single together, and we'd set up a concert. We sat deciding what our tour would be called and came up with the name 'The Grey Diamond Tour'. I would be Andrew's guest singer and speaker, and we would sing a song together. It all felt real, exciting and possible we believed in everything that we said. It was true that Andrew and I had just met but never the less here we were talking about how our lives could be very much entwined as we went forward on a path together.

We were finally trying to fall asleep at about five or six am, but just as we would be about to drop off something else would occur to one or the other of us. We just had such a great connection, and we could not let sleep rob us of even a minute.

In the morning, we all got up for a delicious cooked breakfast courtesy of Mum. Once we had filled our bellies, we all got ready and booked a taxi to the radio studio.

The two-hour show went well, and it flew by. Afterwards, I had set up a meet and greet. People who wanted to meet Andrew and watch the trailer for the documentary.

After my sleepless night, I was struggling to keep my eyes open, and the hall we had hired out was echoing which made it hard for me to hear what was being said clearly. I decided that I better leave them in Mum's capable hands and jumped on the bus home.

I had a feeling Andrew would worry about my sudden disappearance as it was a bit strange me not coming back so I sent him a text to say I would see him later apologising to have left so abruptly. He replied straight back to me saying that he had been worried but was glad I was ok. I explained about my tiredness, and how it affected me, and it was nice, for once to know that here was someone who genuinely understood what I was saying.

When I woke up from my catnap, they were all back at the house. It sounded like the gathering had been a success.

After another lovely dinner with everyone, I asked Andrew if he wanted to watch movies in my room. Now I wanted to spend as much time with him as possible as I knew that he would be leaving the following morning. We made some popcorn and headed upstairs. I knew it was a little rude leaving Paul and Theresa with my parents, but I really did not want to waste a moment of being with Andrew. I was being selfish – I wanted him all to myself.

As we sat watching TV with the lights off and just the glow from the screen, I was beginning to get butterflies in my tummy. That was a feeling that I had not had for the longest time, and I realised that I liked this guy a lot. I was sitting as close as possible to him without sitting on him. I felt relief wash over me as it was becoming clear now that he felt the same way about me.

I wanted him to kiss me, so I decided to make it as visible as possible. I screwed up my courage and asked him boldly "You want to kiss me, don't you?" He smiled and laughed and said, "Yes". I was thinking in my head "Just do it!" And then he did.

We sat cuddled up watching the films and just appreciated the time that we had together. I didn't want the evening to end. We tried to stay awake talking as long as possible but after a sleepless night the night before we were both exhausted and we both fell asleep.

I woke up early to get Paul, Andrew and Teresa into a taxi to London Heathrow Airport. They were flying to

Norway where they were going to produce the soundtrack that Andrew had written for the film.

As they drove away, I had no idea if I would hear from Andrew again. I was trying to keep calm and had to force myself not be the first person to message. When I received Andrews's text later that day, I was so glad that I felt quite emotional:

"I can't stop thinking about the last two days I spent with you. I could have just spent time with you all day and night talking, watching movies, making each other laugh, and besides all that I just have to say I feel like I have met a unique and beautiful person in you! I know we will keep in touch and see what happens! I do believe we met for a huge purpose."

I had a smile as broad as the Indian Ocean. I had heard those cliched stories before about people who had known very soon after meeting someone that they would be with them forever. I was astonished to realise that I was saying to myself I'm going to marry this man!

The next few weeks, were a whirlwind of mutual adoration, admiration and excitement about where this adventure would go. It felt like Andrew had left my life as quickly as he came into it, but he had definitely left a print on my heart. I knew we were going to try and see if we could make it work. We both hoped it was in God's plan for us to stay together.

We both carried on our lives, I worked on the radio shows, and Andrew was singing most weeks with his band. We would text each other every five minutes, sharing every little thing what we were up to. Every question we asked each other was a tick in the box. What was nice though as we both said that if either of us were ever unwell or just feeling very fatigued, then neither of us would be upset if plans had to be cancelled. We both knew that feeling of having to say no or drop out where our sometimes-precarious health was concerned, and we would never make the other feel bad over any missed dates for anything.

We quizzed each other imagining scenarios that we might face once we were officially together and we discussed how we would deal with whatever we faced.

Andrew put forward his scenario: "Ok, so I'm doing a concert or show, and you're, of course, backstage enjoying it!! The show is over, and I have fans to greet and meet, do you stay by my side while I do this, or get upset because you want to leave? (But so that you know you will always come first with things like that)".

I loved every minute of our conversations, and we were entirely on the same page, no question of that. He told me he had written a song about me, to put all his feelings and emotions about us on paper.

What an amazing thing to have been said!

I knew we were potentially taking a big risk, but there was no doubt that it felt right. In a swift decision, because I had decided that if this was going to stand a chance of working, we needed to be able to spend some more time together, so I suggested travelling to New

York to meet him. It was entirely out of my comfort zone, and I was going by blind faith. To my delight, he was more than happy to spend some more time together, and I just could not wait.

I knew the trip was not going to be a problem in respect to us spending too much time together, as we always had so much to say. The problem was going to be leaving Andrew behind at the end of it, and that was going to be very hard.

On the 18th August, I booked a flight to New York, arranging with Andrew that he would meet me there for a few days. I knew we were taking a significant risk, but it felt so right.

While Andrew and I were falling in love very quickly, I still was committed to my radio show and my part in getting people to share their experiences. Every week Andrew would manage to wake up at 7 am EST time to listen to my show, and I loved his support. Although my show was very much a talk show, we did play music too. I would play songs that were relevant to Andrew and me. Only we would know it was for us. One of our favourites was the "All of Me" by John Legend.

A slightly awkward moment came when my Radio Manager told me that all use of the Internet was recorded to make sure any presenter did not misuse the Internet. Suddenly we had the horrific realisation that all our mushy and romantic conversations were being read. I was so embarrassed and immediately stopped the dialogue with Andrew. We confined ourselves to the use of my personal mobile and WhatsApp.

Ticking Off Boxes

In September, I had my regular MRI scan to check that there was no further recurrence from my intraventricular atrial meningioma. The wait for the results is always a bit worrying, but I was hopeful. On the 22nd September, it was confirmed there was no sign of a tumour. It showed I still had a lot of scarring and I was, therefore, was advised to stay on seizure medication. I was told I did not need to have another scan for two years and that was great news.

When I looked back, I was slowly a ticking off boxes that I could move away from. I know the likelihood of my vision coming back to normal was now slim to none, but I always said, never say never. My hearing sensitivity was a big problem and really triggered my panic attacks, and Dr Minhas said he would set up an appointment with the hearing specialist to see if this might be the result of the surgery or if it was just due to anxiety.

I had my hearing examination at St George's in the Tinnitus/Hyperacusis Clinic. It took about 4 hours for the testing and then I went to see a specialist who handed me a diagnosis of hyperacusis. She said I had increased sensitivity to environmental sounds and that this would explain why I just could not tolerate noise. She said that this was not uncommon because of brain surgery. She would send a letter to my GP and would discuss a possible course of action for me.

Once I finally had my appointment about my hearing, the doctor suggested I use hearing generators. To be honest, I was not really feeling that. But I said I would try it.

Back to Google to see what generators are: This is what I found out:

Hyperacusis (or hyperacusis) is a debilitating hearing disorder characterised by an increased sensitivity to certain frequencies and volume ranges of sound (a collapsed tolerance to usual environmental sound). One type of treatment is using special noise generators. They look like standard hearing aids, but there is a constant hissing noise to build up a person tolerance.

I took my generators away with me and was told to try them for 2 weeks and then come back to say to the specialist how I was getting on. When I first put the hearing aids in, they made my ears itch like crazy, and they hurt my skin. I tried to tolerate them, but I was getting headaches. I didn't feel this would work for me.

More charities were getting in touch to ask us to promote their events. A few to mention amongst others are The National Brain Appeal 'Pyjama Party' and Brain Tumour Research 'Wear A Hat Day' and much more. We always loved taking part and dressing up in the studio to send photos and donate to the organizers what we had collected.

Because I had had so many medical appointments through the last five years, I decided to email all my specialists and asked if I could interview them about their expertise in treating brain tumours.

I was particularly interested in talking with the 'Sister of Eye Day Care at the Eye Unit at Croydon University Hospital'. She talked about how often they see brain tumours when people come in for routine check-ups. It was surprising to hear that there are so many things that could be found by examining the eyes. I mentioned my partial blindness and asked if she thought there was any chance that the situation would improve. The sister did give me a glimmer of hope telling me that finding new cures were being discovered all the time and that work was going on all the time to try to find fixes for things. That was very encouraging, and I felt a lump in my throat as I contemplated my gleam of hope.

Before I knew it, the year had just flown by, and it was December 2nd. I was packed and ready to go to New York and see Andrew. I was thrilled but anxious at the same time. It was a big deal for me that I was taking this trip alone. After my 10-hour flight, I arrived at JFK airport. I had got on a shuttle bus to the hotel, and the driver told me that it was likely to be a while as it was rush hour in the city. Even so, I had no idea it would take three hours to get there! I was the last passenger to get off. Andrew was already at the hotel after his own long coach trip from Providence. I felt terrible that he had waited over 3hrs for me.

My heart was pounding as I walked through the lobby of the Intercontinental Hotel and over to the check-in desk. The light was very dim, and I couldn't see that well. There was a man about three meters away from me, and as nobody else was there, I guessed it was Andrew. He looked different, and I began to panic a bit. It had only been four months since we saw each other face to face, but 'oh boy' did he look different. As I steeled myself, the man walked away. For a split second, I thought 'Yikes, he's gone'. Then I saw Andrew. He was sitting on the lobby sofa behind. There was the man I remembered! A big cheesy smile lit up my face.

I picked up the hotel key and walked to Andrew and said hello. We were both clearly shy, and he put his hand out and led me to the elevators. As we waited for a lift to the 6th floor with our luggage, we were smiling. I thought I would break the ice and gave him a big hug and a big kiss. We got to our room, and to my delight, we found that we had been upgraded to the Deluxe King Room. We had a lovely view over Times Square. Holding hands, we both just flopped onto the bed with relief that we had made it and we were together again.

We decided to get up and go into the city for a drink. We both had no idea where to go, and we went to the first bar we saw. We sat talking and enjoying each other's company. We didn't stay too long. We went back to the hotel and raided the mini bar and ate the complimentary chocolate and refreshments from our room fridge. We rested on the bed listening to Andrew's iPhone playlist that he had put together with all our favourite tracks.

The following day I was wide awake at 5 am as I was still running on British time. Andrew would have liked more sleep. To make up for waking him up so early, I ordered breakfast in the room. I think that smoothed things over. The meals are so big and full of sugar. Yummy.

Looking out of the window, it seemed so lovely and sunny, but I knew it would be cold. I could see the steam spiraling up from the grates along the street. It was an iconic New York sight. We wrapped up warm and headed to The Empire State Building and travelled right up to the top. We were rewarded with magnificent views over New York. It was like the scene from 'Sleepless in Seattle' with Meg Ryan and Tom Hanks. We were two people from entirely different worlds, but it worked, and I really loved him, and I knew that he loved me too.

I had organised for us to meet a friend called Rosalie and her husband on the 4th whom I had initially met on my Aunty M Brain Tumours Facebook Page two years earlier. Rosalie had been through her own brain tumour battles but was one of the bubbliest people I've ever come across. She has an incredible sense of humour and makes me laugh so much. I was looking forward to Andrew and Rosalie meeting each other.

We had made plans to meet in Times Square by the big Christmas tree in the center. But I hadn't realised that New York was on shutdown as Mariah Carry was arriving to turn the Christmas lights on in the city. It was absolutely packed. Finding each other was going to be next to impossible, we very nearly gave up and were about to give up when by some miracle we saw each other.

We piled into a taxi to take us to a nice Italian restaurant that Rosalie and her husband had been going to for years. As we were driving past all the crowds heading towards the big Christmas tree, a nun came to the window, and Rosalie told the sister we were brain tumour survivors. In a surreal moment, she gave us all a pendant with the Virgin Mary on and blessed us all.

We finally got to the restaurant and sat down. We were left with no uncertainty that we were to be treated by Rosalie's husband who wanted to pay for everything. The connection between Rosalie and her husband was electric; they bounced off one another and were entirely in sync. I couldn't help hoping that is how I want to be with my husband one day.

After our meal, we wished Rosalie and her husband farewell and went on our way. It was only 8 pm, so we decided to go to the 250 Fifth Rooftop Bar. I had read about it before I came to New York. They gave blankets to everyone as it was freezing outside. The blankets were bright red, and when you put the hoods up, everyone looked like Little Red Riding Hood. I managed to get Andrew to put his hood up and quickly took a selfie before he took it off. It was not a look that went with his usual cool persona.

After a beautiful evening, we went back to our hotel. It was our last night in New York, and I felt sick knowing after that day was going to really put a strain on our relationship. We had no plans for when we would meet again. There was no way we could, while Andrew was doing the film that had no deadline yet.

After what felt like the perfect time together, I felt we had to take a step back, and I suggested maybe we should take a break from the pressure as boyfriend and girlfriend, and that we should just be friends, great friends. It could take over a year for Andrews film to be sorted and I was in no position to up and leave home and live in Rhode Island. I knew it was a big ask, I loved him and hoped he would understand and agree.

His response was: "I love you with all I have, and I don't want to lose what we have built, but it makes sense what you are saying. I will accept a break or however you want to put it in your words. I'd rather have you as a friend for now than lose you altogether. I can't imagine losing someone I love so much completely. You are an amazing woman, and I hope I am the man you are supposed to be with. I think I could be perfect for you. I guess it's just not now. I love you, Claire...I really do, and I only want what's best for you."

I headed back to London and hoped the wait between now and when I met with Andrew again would be fast and not too hard. I needed to keep as busy as possible.

Charity of The Month

I decided that I needed to hit the ground running. I contacted Tina Boden who had really helped me in the beginning when I set up Aunty M Brain Tumours. She is a constant connector, bringing people and organisations together to make a difference, a real problem solver.

I explained I was going to start a Charity of The Month Campaign for my radio show. I wanted her help to put a letter together that I would send to 12 charities that support brain tumour patients and research centers. It would be the 12 Charities that I had connected with on my social platforms. Now I wanted to use my radio show as a voice for them.

I showed Tina the list of charities I wanted to reach out too. She loved the idea and went away to put a letter together. I knew Tina would do a great job as she is as passionate about raising awareness and raising funds for brain tumour research as I am.

Dear……….

Aunty M Brain Tumours: Charity of the Month

I would like to invite (Charity Name) to be Aunty M Brain Tumours Charity of the Month in (Month and Year).

You may have heard of Aunty M Brain Tumours through social media or your connections within the brain tumour community. I was diagnosed in 2008, when I was 25, with a brain tumour finding myself being operated on 3 days after diagnosis.

3 years after my surgery I set up Aunty M Brain Tumours as a feel-good Facebook group to help others that had also been affected by a brain tumour, ensuring they had a lifelong support network not just help when they were being treated.

A year later, with 400 people in the Facebook group, I set up Aunty M Brain Tumours website www.auntymbraintumours.co.uk and things have just grown from there.

Now with a published book, A Brain Tumour's Travel Tale, a weekly radio show on Croydon Radio and with over 10000 people worldwide per month engaging with Aunty M Brain Tumours, I want to develop further the support and help that I give.

Over the coming months, Aunty M Brain Tumours will establish a social enterprise that allows me to raise brain tumour awareness and support people affected by a brain tumour, whether a patient, family, carer or friend without becoming a charity.

It is important to me to promote the work that charities are doing to support brain tumour patients, their families, friends and carers as well as looking at the research that is taking place worldwide that will make a difference for brain tumour patients of the future.

Aunty M Brain Tumours Charity of the Month will:

Receive social media promotion through all Aunty M networks
Receive website promotion on the Aunty M site

183

Be interviewed on our Thursday lunchtime show on Croydon Radio sometime during their charity of the month period.

If you feel that being Aunty M's charity of the month would be beneficial to your charity, please send an email to me at auntymbraintumours@gmail.com

I look forward to hearing from you.
Yours sincerely

Claire Bullimore

I put together a list of the charities, and we sent the letter off. I was thrilled when they all came back positive, and all wanted to be involved. I picked a charity for each month, and we were set:

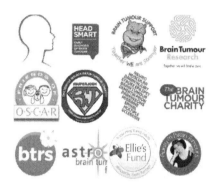

January – Brainstrust

February - Headsmart

March - Brain Tumour Support

April - Brain Tumour Research

May – Friends of O.S.C.A. R

June - The Joshua Wilson Brain Tumour Charity

July - The National Brain Appeal

August - The Brain Tumour Charity

September – Brain Tumour Research South Yorks (BTRS)

October - Astro Brain Tumour Fund

November - Ellie Fund

December – Aunty M Brain Tumours

Christmas had arrived before I could turn around, and I was looking forward to my brother Ian and his girlfriend spending three weeks with my family and me. I hadn't spent Christmas with Ian in the UK for over 6yrs. We had a lovely few weeks and lots of food and drink with friends and family.

On the 31st December, I started writing a New Year

To Do List:

Radio Show Interviews
Update Website
Produce Audio Book
Start Charity of The Month Shows
Plan A Book Tour around the UK
Start 2nd Book
Start A Lifestyle Blog
Make YouTube Channel
Record Some Songs for YouTube
I will NOT let ANXIETY hold me back

When Big Ben rang at 00:00 on the 1st January 2014, it was time to put my action plan together. My first task was to set up a UK book tour. I wanted to meet the people who had been connecting with my Aunty M Brain Tumours social media platforms over the last three years. I really wanted it to start over the summer through to December. I didn't have a clue how I would do it or how I would fund it.

I had to think hard about what to do, and so I emailed Tina Boden again and asked if she could help me and she suggested that I start a crowdfunding campaign to raise funds. Tina gave me the contact for her colleague, Lorraine, who could mentor me. Lorraine had undertaken crowdfunding campaigns for other people. At that time, I must admit that I had absolutely no idea what crowdfunding was. I went straight to my go-to reference point - the Internet, to look it up.

Google says "Crowdfunding is the practice of funding a project or venture by raising monetary contributions from a large number of people. Crowdfunding is a form of crowdsourcing and of alternative finance."

That looked absolutely great and exactly what I was looking for. I got in touch with Lorraine and explained to her what I wanted to do. Lorraine went away to put a strategy together. I was looking forward to seeing how this would work, but I was also worried that I wouldn't be able to meet the target and even worse, nobody would want to help me. That's right Claire, 'way to be optimistic!'

We decided the best website to put my campaign on was 'UK Crowdfunder'. The rules are that I had to raise the money within 28 days, if I didn't reach the target, then all money went back to the people who pledged. That is something else that is part of crowdfunding, is to give gifts to the people who pledge.

There is no guarantee I would reach the target, and you must put a lot of finance in first in preparation and to get the campaign up and running. It is probably not the most comfortable or easy route, but if it worked, it would be perfect to make my plans come together.

I reached out to my social media platforms and asked people if they would come to my book signings. I was not sure if anyone would be interested in the slightest, I was asking people to buy my books and was not at all confident that they would want to, I hoped I had in some way supported others on my websites, and they would want to come to meet me.

Thankfully, when I asked for it, the support from people was incredible. I felt fortunate to have such an incredible network of friends and supporters of Aunty M Brain Tumours. I then looked for where everyone lived to plan the route, I would take around the country.

After planning the route, I needed to find venues. I reached out to the brain tumour charities and asked if I could join their support groups. Their help was tremendous. I was so grateful.

On my tour, I was also able to stay with friends and family, and I would only need to stay at a few hotels. I put together days and times spanning between July and December.

My route was planned:

York -BTRS

Leeds – Brainstrust

Preston – Katy Holmes

Manchester – Brainstrust and Dawn and SuperJosh

Edinburgh – Brainstrust

Glasgow – Brainstrust

Sheffield – Brainstrust

Derby – Brainstrust

Birmingham – Brain Tumour Support

Bedford – Joss Searchlight

St Austell – Brain Tumour Support

Plymouth – Brain Tumour Support

Portsmouth – Brainstrust

Brighton – Brainstrust

Cardiff – Brainstrust

Kent – East Kent Brain Tumour Support

Croydon – Home Party

I wanted to continue with my weekly radio show, and I had to plan that around managing my own ongoing health problems, including hospital appointments and dealing with chronic fatigue. It was a big project, but I was determined to do it.

Once the locations were sorted, I put rewards together for the people who pledged. Most of the gifts had a 'Have A Cuppa' theme. I always liked to think tea, or any beverage could be a comfort or a pick-me-up when times get hard for people. They could come online on Facebook or Twitter pages and have a chat with others who understood their worries or frustrations. The 'Have A Cuppa' theme was also for celebrating the good things such as excellent results for MRI scans or finishing any kind of treatment.

I had also decided I would make small goodie bags for everybody who came to the book signings as a thank you. I knew my Art and Design classes would come in useful one day I thought as I admired my work. Eat your heart out, Blue Peter! I made see-through bags that looked a bit like the triangle shaped tea bags. They had gifts in them that were associated with me and Aunty M Brain Tumours. They included a brain tumour awareness ribbon brooch, teabags and more.

Once they were in production, Lorraine put a spreadsheet together with what I would need and how much the book tour would cost. She said I would need to raise £5,200, but she would walk me through the campaign and getting publicity.

Once we had the figure that I was reaching for, I had to do a 3-minute video for the crowdfunding page explaining who I was and what it was I needed help with.

I had to laugh at myself, as it took me about 20 takes to get the video right. I just kept forgetting what I was saying, and that was even when I had it written down! Not the most comfortable thing for a person who has had brain surgery or is partially blind and can hardly see the words on the page.

In April I had my video ready to put on YouTube, and it was getting some interest. Once that was sorted the crowdfunding page was set to go live in May. I knew I had another few months to make up the goodie bags and build up momentum for the live crowdfunding campaign

Radio Gaga

I continued to work on the radio show giving brain tumour awareness the publicity I wanted it to have, and I was invited to be an advocate for the brain tumour community at the Houses Of Parliament about the 'The Saatchi Bill'. The Saatchi Bill was all about patients being able to have a 2nd opinion on treatments rather than the current situation where if that was what a patient wanted, they really did not have any option except to go private after the first diagnosis had been given by the NHS. I wanted my friends, and others who are suffering from cancer or other long-term illnesses, to be able to say to their doctor "can you do anything, what are the treatments available, is there anything new that I can try?' and know that their doctor would point them in the right direction if that were appropriate.

All these opportunities were helping me keep my mind on what I was doing and keeping me from missing Andrew so much. It was impossible not to miss him though. We had been able to speak on and off and try to keep a connection. It was getting harder, and the idea that our plans might not come to fruition was becoming a very painful possibility.

We were always checking in on each other to make sure each other was doing ok, and we both seemed to be stable, medically. Andrew was having physiotherapy as he was still weak on one side. He was still performing on stage although there appeared to be a hold on the film, which was a little discouraging for both of us, we just kept hold of all we had discussed and reassured each other. It was all we could do.

In March my 'The Charity of the Month' had been going great. My goal was to give the charities a voice to explain why they were trying to get money from people. I felt it was important for the public to meet the people who set up a charity and what their personal experiences were. When people start posting messages to the world, wanting their donations, it was obvious why and how important people's contribution was going to be.

In January, my first Charity of The Month was Brainstrust. I interviewed Dr Helen Bulbeck, one of the Founders and Director of Brainstrust. She explained that in 2004 her daughter Meg who was 18 at the time was diagnosed with a brain tumour.

Helen recollected how A and E had phoned her up to say her daughter Meg was in hospital following a possible seizure. To Helen's surprise, this was not the first time Meg had had a seizure. She had not told anyone - she just didn't want to worry her mum. Helen and her husband headed to the hospital and Helen had thoughts running through her head wondering if Meg's drink had been drugged while she had been out the night before.

It took a few weeks before the doctors could diagnose Meg. Sadly, it was a brain tumour. They had told them that the tumour was a grade 2. Helen remembers that she was in absolute shock and utterly speechless. They had no idea where to find support because, back then, there wasn't any.

They could see there was some research being worked on but no engagement and support for how they felt and what they could find that would help Meg. Helen felt like they were in a black hole and really struggling.

After doing their own research, they were told there was a treatment available in America, and if they could raise funds, they could take Meg over to Boston and be treated. The cost for the operation in Boston was over £35,000. Meg and her family were able to put a fundraiser together through Meg's 6th form college and were looking to raise £20,000. They had 18 months to raise funds before Meg needed to go for the treatment and amazingly and miraculously people raised £70,000.

Meg had her operation, and it was a success. They still had £35,000 left. They felt Meg's story was a very positive story, so they decided to put the rest of the funds into setting up a trust to help other people and make sure they knew where to find support. They didn't want people to feel as lost as they had felt the day, they were told Meg had a brain tumour.

And so Brainstrust was born. It quickly became a place that as Helen had hoped people used as the first port of call to direct people towards the help and support, they needed. They started setting up meetups around the U.K where patients, carers or family and friends could meet up and have a free meal and meet others who understood precisely what they were going through.

I had the pleasure of joining one of their meetups in London in 2012 and met Helen and Meg. It was fantastic. There were around 12 people there, all at different stages of diagnosis or recovery. At first, I was nervous as I hadn't personally met anybody else in my position. I had connected with people on my websites, but I had not met anyone face to face at that point. The atmosphere was very relaxed and was at a time in the day where the restaurant was not too busy. I personally would not have been able to go to the event if it had been held at a noisy time of day.

I asked Helen what she hoped the future for Brainstrust was and asked her to tell us what they were working on other than the meetups and the website which is full of information. Helen said they would continue to add to the information available on the site and keep building up awareness.

They wanted to meet the needs of patients. One thing they knew was a very common problem was the overwhelming fatigue that people experienced and that controlled people's lives, and so the charity had set up support groups for that. They wanted to listen to the public and meet their needs.

I had a brownie point as I had asked my Facebook page followers what they did to help with fatigue. There was so much feedback; Helen was able to put all that feedback towards the upcoming support group sessions that she was setting up.

I looked forward to following up on the work Brainstrust were doing and as a brain tumour survivor myself, I was so grateful for their dedication and the way that they were really listening to the patients' needs.

My February charity of the month was Headsmart, which isn't quite a charity as it is more of a campaign run by The Brain Tumour Charity. The campaign is an on-going project and so is very important.

Headsmart was set up from the concerns of families and healthcare professionals about the prolonged time it was taking for children and teenagers with a brain tumour to be diagnosed. The campaign includes a symptoms card, which tells a person the warning, signs to look out for.

I interviewed James Walsh who was the Policy and Campaigns Manager for Headsmart. One of his roles was to get as many schools and doctors to have the cards available for people to take away so that they became familiar with the signs.

When I asked why he joined the charity, my heart sank as he explained how his mother had died from brain cancer in 2012 when he was only in his twenties. No matter how many people I speak to about losing a loved one, my heart just drops when it is a mother or father when the son or daughter is still so young.

I was so grateful that he felt able to share his experience with me and that he was using the experience in a very positive way."

In March my Charity of the Month was Brain Tumour Support. I had the pleasure of interviewing Julie Liddle. A mother and wife whom I had initially met in 2012 via Aunty M Brain Tumours. When we first met Julie had only recently had her diagnosis. I was so happy to see that now she had become a Cornwall/Devon Brain Tumour Support Worker.

In 2011 Julie was doing a degree at university, a tough enough task in itself but she was also suffering from terrible headaches. Julie thought that the headaches were stress related. As the headaches got worse, she decided that she needed to go to the Doctor. The doctor put it down to her suffering from the very vague diagnosis - chronic headaches. Julie and her husband were not happy with the diagnosis, and they wanted a second opinion. They went private, but again the diagnosis was chronic headaches and nothing more.

Then one-night Julie almost collapsed, and her husband was determined that enough was enough, Julie needed a scan. She went back to her GP, and a CT scan was ordered. It turned out that Julie's 'chronic headaches' were actually due to a 5cm brain tumour, a posterior fossa meningioma.

Within a few weeks, Julie was booked in for brain surgery. They were able to remove some of the tumour but not all of it. They would have to keep an eye on it, and if it grew too big, they would do some radiotherapy.

After her own recovery and feeling much stronger, Julie went to find support near her and came across Brain Tumour Support. Starting as a guest and finding the support groups very helpful, Julie soon became a Brain Tumour Support Worker in the Cornwall and Devon area. The idea is to create a friendly place for people to share their experiences and meet others who were on the same journey as they were. It is entirely free, and there are always cakes and refreshments. There are usually around 12 people in a group. The charity also gets speakers to come in and speak to the group. They have a lady who can pick people up and drop them off if it is hard for them to travel. There are support groups in Staffordshire, Shropshire, Walsall, Wolverhampton, Birmingham, Warwickshire, Worcestershire, Herefordshire, Gloucestershire, Bristol, Somerset, Hampshire, Dorset, Devon and Cornwall

They are always friendly and very welcoming. I was looking forward to seeing more of the work they would do in the future.

In April, Lorraine helped me get some publicity out there for the build-up to the crowdfunding campaign in the shape of The Wright Stuff TV Show, where Richard Madeley was presenting and talking to a famous Singer called Kerry Ellis. She was promoting her own crowdfunding campaign for a music tour. My project was mentioned referring to other people, like me, who have turned to crowdfunding to raise funds.

It was my first ever mention on the national TV programme. That was pretty pants wettingly exciting. That got the ball rolling, and within a week I was mentioned in a few local newspapers and on national blogs. Lots of the brain tumour charities around the UK were helping to get the word out there.

I think my favorite of all the businesses that were supporting me, and my campaign was Croydon Radio. The managers, Tracey and Tim, were amazingly supportive. It has been an absolute pleasure to be a part of the Croydon Radio team since January 2013. The radio directors had been nothing but supportive of the brain tumour community and showed it by giving us a voice on the Brain Tumour Thursday Show. They asked other shows to mention my campaign and set up a banner on the main website.

On April 27th, my campaign went live, and by 25th May it was all over. It felt like it was one of the fastest and at the same time one of the slowest months I had ever had. But, 28 days of working our butts off, we did it. Because of people's generosity and support for the Book

Tour, it was possible to go ahead. We reached 110% funding, Raising a fantastic £5,710.

That was all sorted, but there was still so much to do. I had 1 month to really promote the book tour and let people know it was happening. I kept a blog via Tumblr so people could see the specific locations I was coming to and when. I couldn't officially promote the times before as there was no guarantee I would reach the crowdfunding target and go ahead with the tour.   Now it was Go, Go, Go.

Although I was sorting out the book tour, there were still hospital appointments to attend. I went to see the hearing specialist again who had diagnosed me initially with hyperacusis. She said because I had not got on very well with the hearing generators, she wanted me to see a specialised CBT hearing therapist. She would refer me to the specialist who was based at the hospital in north London. I was happy with that idea and waited for an appointment. letter.

While I was back on the waiting list, I had lots going on. I was only a month away from the book tour. I was invited to be a guest at a street party that was taking place for a brain tumour research fundraising event and had also been invited to an annual Amber Ball in London set up by Brain Tumour Research. It was such a beautiful evening, and everyone was dressed up in their finest. The women were all wearing ball gowns, and the men all looked so smart in their formal clothing. This was an event that had many wealthy people in attendance, and nearly a million pounds was raised. AMAZING.

I really did appreciate the opportunities I was being given and loved every minute of it. I always wished Andrew could have been part of it as he is himself, is a walking miracle after surviving three brain tumours, and I know that he would have loved to share these opportunities with me.

I went home that night and wrote a letter to Andrew:

Dear Mr Reis,

I just wanted to say; I love you very much. I thought I'd write you this because maybe you'll keep it and one day we'll look back and say…. It was worth the wait. I will always hold on to the feeling I had from your time in the UK and our time in New York and our conversations. I do hope we will be together one day.   In my heart I know it will happen and all the distance we have now will become a distant memory. I know we are busy, and you have a lot to resolve. I know it is not easy on you waiting for things to fall into place but, it will soon. I honestly believe that.

I know it is my Birthday in 2 weeks on Thursday, and I was trying hard to put something together to see you that weekend, but it is Mother's Day over here on that Sunday too, so I need to be homed that week. Probably just as well as if I had done something mad and impulsive, you might have told me off about doing it - lol. Perhaps we'll get to do something in May. I know there is going to be a bunch of hurdles we will have to jump including our friendship, probably because of misunderstandings or just because I am very impatient. However, I am learning to be less impatient every day.

Claire (Miss B)

His reply was:

Miss B,

I love you very much too. I hope and wish everything we ever spoke about together does come together, even though at this time things are busy and hectic for the both of us. It won't always be this hectic, but I guess this is just the calm before the storm, and when all is settled, we will come out of it stronger and better than before! I too still hold on to my trip there and meeting you as one of the very best experiences in my life!! As well as New York and our time spent there was amazing! I do have to say thank you for your undeniable patience with me at this time in my life which is extremely tough as you know, but you have been extraordinarily patient and kind and helpful to me and words cannot describe how appreciative I am.

Mr R.

In these messages, I realised we were in another place in our life where we had said goodbye to the romantic relationship but not our friendship. It was the time we went our own ways and what would be would be. But for now, we were officially just friends. Great friends.

Book Tour Time

1st July, it was day 1 of my Book Tour, and I was heading to York to join the Brain Tumour Research South Yorkshire Group (BTRS). It was a 5hr drive from London, and my mum was my chauffer for this one. We stocked up with sweets and water for the car and packed our bags for a 3-night trip away. It was a kind of going on holiday feel, although I could not help but feel a bit nervous along with the excitement.

We arrived in the afternoon at the hotel. It was also where the first meetup would be. I had the pleasure of meeting Tina Boden again and Rachel Wilson who was the Charity Manager from BTRS. It was their first support group in this area, so it was a new experience for both of us. 30mins into the meet-up, nobody had turned up. I started to feel rattled. Was this going to happen at every meeting? Oh boy, I hoped not. This could be a disaster.

Rachel told me that they had a feeling this would happen as they hadn't done a meeting in that area before and most people from around there would have been in the habit of going to Leeds for the meetup which was to be my next event in two days time.

The following morning, we woke up and packed up ready to drive on to Leeds. I had no idea how beautiful York was, it was so picturesque, and the scenery was so impressive. Sometimes when you live in the London bubble, you don't realise how lovely the rest of England is. We drove away from York and went to Leeds. We were booked into the Crown Plaza as that was where the meeting would be the following day.

Tina and Rachel had come early to meet me and set up the meeting room. I had a table set up with my books laid out and available to buy, and I had my goodie bags ready to give to everybody who came along.

I didn't really know what to expect, and Tina was great at reassuring me and keeping me calm and just making sure I was set to go. I had put a PowerPoint presentation together with a quick insight into my personal experience.

As people started turning up, I was in shock at how many people there were. It was, no doubt, a fantastic turnout. I recognised many people who I had met through my websites, and I was so appreciative that they had taken the trouble to join me.

I shared my story with them and answered any questions they had about my experience, hoping that might help them if they were at the beginning of diagnosis.

My heart would sink when I'd meet people who were clearly struggling with processing the diagnosis, and I hoped I could encourage people with how far I had come.

I had bought an empty book a kind of visitor's book for people to sign if they wanted to leave a message after the meeting. I wasn't sure if anyone would sign in it. After the meeting and having a lovely time, I was ready for a nap. It was very exhausting, and for a change, I could tell that lots of people here knew exactly how I felt as they had their own trials and similar experience.

As I lay in bed, I was reading through the comments that had been left in my 'visitors' book'. They were so encouraging.

"To my Aunty M, who was there when I needed to find you. Part of our family FOREVER - Claire Dent."

"Thank you for the lovely talk tonight. We can relate to everything you mentioned. Very inspirational - Matt & Jo."

"Claire, you are truly inspirational to so many. Keep up the great work - Lisa Brydon."

"You are an inspiration, great talk and such passion - Lesley & Andrew Sharman."

My heart was full of gratitude.

The following day it was time to pack up and drive on to Preston, to meet Paula Holmes, mother of Katie and the founder of Katie Holmes Trust. I had heard about the Trust a few years earlier. It was a charity dedicated to raising awareness of pediatric brain tumours and raising money to fund the research in memory of 10-year-old Katy Holmes.

North of the border next, it was time to take the train to Scotland and join the Brainstrust meetups in Edinburgh and Glasgow. I had never been to Scotland before. I was blown away by how beautiful it was.

Once back to London on the 17th Andrew had his scheduled 6-month MRI scan. I was nervous to hear his results, but I was staying positive that he would be given the all clear. To my utter devastation, he wasn't. The scan showed he had another malignant tumour.

The blood drained from my face. I went white. I felt sick. I crouched down on the floor. I felt helpless; all I wanted to do was give him a big hug. I could hear the disappointment in his voice. It was terrible news.

Physically he had been feeling a lot stronger from his physio and from keeping fit. He said he would be going back on the Tramadol pill but was determined to keep working as he needed to earn money.

I thought to myself, how can this be? He beat cancer and had been cancer free for so long. Why was this happening? How naive had I been? I really thought he was cancer free and he would never have to fight cancer again. I felt because he had a grade 3 and not a grade 4, he would be ok unless it went to a grade 4, right? I had so many unanswered questions in my mind.

Andrew was ready to fight again, he had no intention of letting cancer beat him. I loved his determination. We knew we were putting this situation into God's hands and prayed he would continue to give Andrew the strength he needed to cope.

I still had lots of meetups to go, and I needed to stay focused. I was looking forward to my next book signing that was in Manchester. Another city I had never been to before. I was able to speak at the Brainstrust meetup, and I was thrilled to see Dawn and Super Josh joined us from the Joshua Wilson Charity.

The next day I head back to London. I wanted to get a gift for Andrew. I was driven down to the music studio in Guildford, and I sang the song Diamonds. I would make sure I messaged him on Monday as I knew that is when he would have treatment and physiotherapy as the medication was suddenly making him feel very weak.

On the 29th I joined a gym and arranged counseling for every Monday. I needed to speak to somebody about me just feeling very low and exhausted and sorry for myself with my health. I didn't feel right about sharing my feelings with anybody. I had mentioned it to Andrew and that I wanted to speak to somebody about how I was struggling with anxiety and feeling very low. He thought it was a great idea and said that he was thinking of doing the same thing. I needed to talk to somebody about what had been going on. I tried to speak about how I was struggling with my emotions and the anxiety I had from being exhausted all the time. They were things

I had to cope with as they weren't going away, and I wanted to get it off my chest. I hoped it would help.

We were in August, and I was finding it helpful speaking with the counsellor. I also joined my local swimming pool to de-stress me.

By the 12th I was back on the road again for the next book signing at the Brainstrust meet-up in Sheffield.

It was lovely to meet more people and sign their books and share a cuppa with everyone. Sharing our own stories was great. So many of us had such similar experiences.

Something I particularly liked to do was speak to the people who were about to have surgery for their tumours. I was glad that I was able to give them some advice on what to expect and things that may help during the recovery. I'd been there, and worn the tee shirt, after all!

My next stop was Derby. It was another beautiful city, with an extraordinary history. Something I had really enjoyed about all my meetings was seeing the different British Cities and recognising all the places I learnt about in my history classes at school. What an amazing history England has. There are so many castles and landcorporals.

After Derby it was Birmingham. I was able to join the 'Brain Tumour Support' groups at the Birmingham Hospital. One of the people in the group said:

"I couldn't put your book down!!! Claire, it's brilliant! It's a good job you tell your readers to go off to make tea because I realised when I got to that point, I'd had been holding my breath! I got to the end of the book and shouted: No don't stop, I want to find out what happens next! We need another book!"

How lovely was that? Wow, I was blushing.

After Birmingham, I was on to Buckinghamshire to meet the founders of the charity Joss Searchlight.

Joss Parkes parents set up the Charity when he sadly lost his life to a brain tumour in 2011. The charity supports other children and their families to give a personal connection and to show them that they are not alone.

August rolled into September, and my next stop was Southampton. Somebody very special to me joined us. His name was Shawn Skinner, a brain cancer patient who had been fighting cancer for many years and been a massive campaigner for raising awareness for brain tumours. He had set up a campaign a few years earlier, called the 'Wear Grey for A Day' that had raised a tremendous amount of money for Brainstrust. His determination and his faith in God are truly recorporalable, and I was so grateful for his friendship and continued support of the brain tumour community.

On the 22nd I joined the Brainstrust meetup in the vibrant city of Brighton for my book signing. As usual, I was blown away by people's warmth, we were our own tribe, people who really understood what each other was going through.

When it was all over, and I had time to think again, I thought how amazing it was to see my dream come to life. It had been 3 months since the start of my book tour, and I had visited 12 Cities so far. I had taken my book and my story to York, Leeds, Edinburgh, Glasgow, Derby, Sheffield, Southampton, Bedford, Birmingham, Brighton, Manchester and Preston.

Every stop made me appreciate the support people gave each other to get through a terribly frightening and heart-wrenching trial. In every place, people had one goal. To KICK ASS and be able to cope with their own journey. They were looking for information and hearing each other's stories. I had met survivors, sufferers and people who had lost a loved one or are looking for a greater understanding of what their loved one was going through.

Next stop Cornwall!

On the 25th of September, my mother drove us to St Austell where I was a guest at the Brain Tumour Support charity event with a book signing. I was thrilled to join Julie Liddle's support group and meet everyone. It was great to put faces to a name.

After the event as I was heading back to London, I read the guest book that people had signed and left messages in. Julie's message was particularly lovely.

"You were one of the first contacts I made on Facebook, which put me in touch with others living in Cornwall. I was delighted when you said you would come to our charity event, it really means a lot. You are such an inspiration". - Julie Liddle.

The messages people were writing really lifted my spirits and confirmed every long and tiring day working on my social media platforms had been so worthwhile.

October rolled into November, and I was heading to another Brainstrust meetup in Cardiff with my mum – SUPERMUM!

Next, it was on to Kent to join the East Kent Brain Tumour support group, set up by Mr and Mrs Middleton. Mr Middleton had been diagnosed with brain cancer and wanted to set up a support group to give a place in his area for people dealing with brain tumours to meet. His family could not find anywhere before that. How sad, that many support groups had been set up by people because they had nowhere else to go, for support.

It was November, and I was coming to the end of my book tour. I joined another Brainstrust meetup in Bournemouth and then headed to the Cotswold's for another book signing in Cheltenham.

What a wonderful way to finish the book tour – arriving in Plymouth to join the opening of the new Plymouth University Research Centre of Excellence, for Brain Tumour Research. There were about 200 people there, and everyone had the same goal - raising awareness and funds for brain tumour research.

Christmas Jingles in my Ears

December had crept up like a Christmas cracker and arrived with a festive 'bang'! The book tour was finished. I put together 'Welcome Home' drinks in Croydon for anyone who wanted to join me. Very kindly my local newspapers shared my celebration and let everyone know that I had just returned from the 6-month book tour. My friend who was the manager of a bar in Croydon allowed me to hire part of it to host the event, and as always, Croydon Radio gave me so much support in raising awareness.

I felt a massive sense of achievement for 2014 - it was an end of term feeling, I was de-mob happy! I was full of gratitude for the people who had supported me. None more so than my book tour sidekick, 'Mum'. She had been beside me all the way and helped me when I was really feeling the tiredness and feeling very overwhelmed when it got noisy. I'm one lucky girl, and I know it. I never take that for granted.

Now Christmas was in full cry, and we were heading for a brand-new year. As I bade 2014 farewell, I was ready for 2015.

In the New Year, I hit the ground running with a new round of hospital appointments. I was being referred to a hearing specialist who was another CBT program specialist. I really needed help with my hearing. It was a huge problem for me. I would be seeing him for some time, and I was keen to know what we would talk about and what strategies we could look at that might help. If I'm honest, I was not optimistic about the appointments, because my hearing was so bad. Anyway, it's a work in progress, so we shall see.

We were into February, and I was going well with my audiobook recording, and I was keeping up with my radio show. It was exhausting, but I was still enjoying it.

I was still being invited to events and campaigns. On the 4th I was at the National Film Theatre after being invited by The Brain Tumour Charity to see the screening of a new documentary. That was followed by a trip to Bristol to give a talk for Brainstrust about being a patron for one of their projects 'Tissue Donor'.

In March I had a referral Letter from my hearing therapist, David Scott. He was aware of my problems and that I had a lot of trouble sleeping without sleep medication. I was glad he recognised the problem I was having and my real need to sleep through the night without a sleep aid.

He sent a referral letter for me to see a 'Sleep Specialist'. Although I was seeing him about my hyperacusis problems, he acknowledged that I had been having sleep problems for years since my surgery. My lousy sleep ability undoubtedly contributed to my anxiety and inability to cope with loud places. Because of the lack of sleep, I would be even more on edge in noisy environments.

Dr Scott wanted the Sleep Specialist to do an examination to rule out anything unusual that might be contributing to my sleep problems. I really was so grateful for him trying to help me.

I was booked for a sleep study at the London Kings Cross hospital that Dr David Scott suggested with advice to be given by a sleep specialist. I stayed overnight and was strapped up with multiple wires that would measure my vital functions and brain waves. It was all very Sci-Fi. I would have to wait a while for the results to be sent to me and given the next plan of action.

On a HUGE plus side, on the 18th June 2015, I had my brain tumour checkup MRI scan. It came back clear! I was VERY pleased about that. I was told I didn't need another scan for 2 years.

A chapter closed, I hoped. I needed a new project to celebrate. I wondered if there was anything I could do with my book or was that a chapter I needed to close as well? My mind clunked into gear and worked overtime, and eventually, I thought, 'What about an audiobook'? An audiobook or kindle. I had been listening to Audible for years. I wasn't sure how much it would cost me or if it was even possible, as I was not a famous author.

After some research online, I realised it would be possible, and like the Kindle books, it was free to put my book on the website but, if a person bought them, I would only get a small amount as a royalty.

Again, money was not my focus, I just needed projects to keep me busy. So, I set myself up.
I tried to record myself from home, reading my book aloud, but I found it impossible not to be distracted. I went to the Croydon radio producers and asked if there was any way I could use the studio when nobody was using it.

As always, they were so helpful and were happy to do that. I planned to do an hour every other day - hopefully it wouldn't take too long. After a month, recording a few chapters at a time, in July my audiobook was available on Audible and iTunes.

The lady who had put me forward to Bella Magazine in 2011 called me. She had seen that I had an audiobook online and that I had been working on Croydon Radio about 'Aunty M Brain Tumours' and said she wanted to cover the story in 'Choice Magazine'. Of course, again I was flattered and did an interview with the magazine and saw it published in the magazine at the end of September.

There was even better news that month when Andrew had his MRI, and the results were fantastic. The chemo tablets had worked, and he was in remission again. We were both looking forward to the next phase of our lives. Not in the same country but watching each other do well and being happy.

Finally, in December, I saw the Sleep Specialist again with the results of my sleep study, Heaven knows why it took so long to speak about it, but at least I was finally seeing somebody. The results showed that I had a PLM index 142 per hour. She felt that I had RLS, Restless Leg syndrome and was going to be put on tablets at night that would relax my legs. It would take a while to make sure I got the tablets that suited me. Another process I had to go through to get it right.

On the Dec 3rd, I had been invited to the opening of the new Portsmouth Centre Of Excellence. Another project set up for Brain Tumour Research. While I was there, I was introduced to a gentleman from the Dr Hadwen Trust. They are the UK's leading non-animal medical research charity.

They had just joined forces with Brain Tumour Research to focus on research but using no animal testing at all. They were setting up a campaign called The Grande Challenge. They needed help with promoting it. I was more than happy to help to raise awareness of it via my radio show and websites.

They were looking to raise £180,000 for a brain tumour research project. I was flattered to be asked to be an ambassador. Of course, I said 'Yes'.

The campaign was called 'The Grand Challenge'. The aim was for people to raise £1,000 in any way they wanted to. I was able to share the project with others on my websites and talk about it on my radio show.

I also got in touch with one of my teachers from my old primary school. He was my history teacher when I was between 8 and 13. He was now the headmaster at Lancing College Preparatory School in Hove. He said he would love to help and take part.

He invited me to speak to the pupils about my experience and to explain why I was raising £1,000.

I had never spoken to such a large audience and had no idea what I would say. It was time to use my PowerPoint skills on the laptop and put together some bullet points for me to use as a prompt. I tried to make it easy to understand and made it child-friendly and not too scary. Because the fundraiser would not be until April, I had plenty of time to prepare it.

On the 23rd of December, I was playing all the best festive Christmas songs and getting in the mood with a special interview with Nicole Phillips and Lorraine Bateman. Nicole was diagnosed with a brain tumour in 2008. She shared her story and told how her life had been changed so drastically and how she has come out fighting - she has a passionate desire to educate doctors about how to diagnose and then deal with people with brain tumours. Lorraine Bateman was going to talk about a 'naked' calendar that Nicole is a part of and explain how she got ladies to strip for charity. The calendar started as an inebriated idea in a pub one night and has now become a reality thanks to the hard work and dedication of some lovely locals from Leighton Buzzard and the surrounding area.

On January 26th I was off to see the sleep therapist again to report on how my sleep had been, and I had to say that it seemed to be better.

In early February I was in a much better place health wise and Andrew, and I were talking a lot more. We were back on track, and it felt nice.

Right at the end of February, I had started talking with a new guy. I know my heart was very much with Andrew, but it really was not possible to make a long-distance relationship work, and Andrew was now seeing another lady. I did like the new guy, and I thought it was worth seeing how things would go.

On February the 29th I flew to Sydney to see my brother Ian and soon to be sister-in-law Phoebe. They were getting married at the end of that month, and I couldn't wait for their wedding in Sydney. I was going to be there throughout March.

It was a lovely holiday, and the wedding was just fantastic. Ian and Phoebe were so happy, and it was a memorable celebration. Near the end of the trip, I started to feel unwell. I just put it down to overdoing it and being fatigued. My legs were painful and aching all the time, especially at night.

We had gone on a trip to Sydney town center. Inexplicably and without warning, I fainted. It took me a little while to realise what happened as I lay on the deck of the river taxi that was taking us down the city river. I had a big bang on my face where I had hit a metal bar when I fell. I felt so silly. Here we go I thought. What's next?

It did put a downer on my trip, and I was conscious that I could not go out so much. When I returned to London on the 1st of April, I went straight to my Sleep Specialist and asked if what had happened was because of the medication.

She put me on a new medication that she said may take a week to get used to and may make me feel dizzy at first. I went away hoping it would be OK and we agreed I would get in contact with her if there were any problems.

While that was going on, I seemed to have 'got my man' and was officially dating. He was kind and took the fact that I sometimes did not feel well, entirely in his stride. I was very honest about my health, and he didn't mind at all. Lucky me.

I was still working on the radio now 1hr a week, still interviewing others and I started seeing my new guy a lot more. We were spending most days together and even went on a few trips around England. I was feeling horrible and not myself, but I tried to soldier on.

On the 25th of April, I was finally speaking at Lancing College Preparatory School in Hove, for Mr Laurent. I was very unsteady and feeling like I was floating on a cloud a lot of the time. I was able to get a lift there, and I did my absolute best to look OK.

It was so lovely to see Mr Laurent. It had been 20yrs since I had seen him. It was brilliant having a walk down memory lane and to revisit the good memories I had of the school that I had been at for so long.

I was so appreciative of the opportunity Mr Laurent had given me.

After a great fundraiser, the school had raised £1,247 in response to the DHT's 'Grand Challenge'. I received a lovely letter from The Dr Hadwen Trust and Mr Laurent.

"Claire has been incredibly brave, and we are extremely grateful to her for her help in publicizing the Grand

Challenge. We are also very grateful to the Lancing College Preparatory School students for their amazing fundraising effort." – Dr Hadwen Trust."

And Mr Alan Laurent had put a nice message on the Charities notice board:

"We are very proud of our students and their efforts. I am particularly proud of Claire. She is a former pupil of mine and, having known her for many years, it is typical of her that she would respond to her condition in this way, with courage and the determination not to let it beat her while raising awareness to help others."

At the end of July, I had come to the conclusion of my time working with Croydon Radio, and I did my last interview. I asked Andrew or as he is known, 'Ace Diamond' if he would be my final interview. Fitted as it was how we had started. It was a sentimental gesture for both of us.

I was worried his documentary would never actually be finished, so I wanted him to have another platform to share his story as a hip-hop artist and a cancer warrior. To share his story to other people going through the devastating trials of cancer.

This was his interview:

Andrew shared his memories of growing up in the projects, or as he calls it 'the hood', he said his family did not have much money and, so he didn't have many opportunities to better himself. He and others always knew he was incredibly talented; it was just trying to find ways to get better known. He was given many opportunities as a hip-hop artist within street music, but those opportunities were not the opportunities he was looking for.

He was about to have a lot of time to think about what direction he was looking to follow, because in 2005 when he was just 25, and at work, he had a grand mal seizure.

He had never had a seizure before and had no idea what was going on. Thankfully he was with one of his sisters.

Both of them were frightened. She called for an ambulance. They confirmed he had had a seizure.

He went to the hospital, and they did an MRI. They found a brain tumour. It was the size of a golf ball.

They wanted to do surgery to remove it, but they said it was not urgent. He was sent home and asked to come back in a few weeks to have surgery.

At surgery, they found a benign tumour and they were able to get it out. He was tumour free and was sent home with a plan for physio to counteract the effects of the surgery.

In 2006 he has diagnosed again with a tumour in the same place, but this time it was a grade 3 cancerous growth. He was scared, and it was a frightening experience but was determined to fight it.

He remembers going into the surgery and all the surgeons seeming to be happy and jolly, and he was thinking 'You guys are crazy'- in a good way. They put him at ease.

After the surgery, they said it was cancerous, but they had got a tumour out. To prevent another tumour growing, he was given chemo pills and radiation.

He had 6 weeks on the pills that he took at home. He then had 6 weeks of radiation.

Once he did that his medical team told him that he could stay on the chemo pills for 5 years and if he had not had a relapse he would be considered to be in remission.

He got past 5 years cancer free and was working towards getting fit again and back to his music. But sadly, he had another recurrence in 2011. He went on more pills and an IV transfusion. He was also told by a head device called Optune. Optune is a wearable, portable device indicated to treat a type of brain cancer called glioblastoma multiforme, but Andrews doctors felt it would help with his Oligodendroglioma.

By the end of 2011, Andrew was cancer free again. It was then that he met the film producer and decided to go back and film the journey he had been on from diagnosis to the present day.

They also joined up with 4 other people who were on the chemo pill. And that was the basis of the documentary 'These Three Words'.

I met Andrew in London in 2013 when he was cancer free again.
I know so many people were listening to Andrew's interview and recognising it as the genuine journey that they or people they knew had gone through.

What was nice was to talk about how he was in remission from his fourth recurrence. He wanted to show how a person could have more determination, reserves of strength and more will than even they realise.

It was so great to tell people that Andrew was in remission and cancer free again. We just prayed for strength to face anything else that would come.

This time, though, it had taken an even more prominent toll on his body. He was now walking with a cane. He was so tired all the time and struggled to do even the basic things.

With my time on the radio over, I needed to think about what my next project would be. I decided it was going to be another book. I also, although I was fond of the new guy I was with, I wasn't fond enough and decided to end that relationship.

People had often asked if I would ever write another book to show what life was like after brain surgery. I was completely up for that and got back to writing. Well, typing.

As the beautiful summer came to an end, I was feeling good. Tired but good. Andrew and I were talking daily and just keeping each other company. We were both around most days while the rest of the world were out and about in the day.

As I wrote my new book, I was still connecting with others through Aunty M Brain Tumours and supporting any campaigns or when any signatures were needed to raise brain tumour funding.

Summer was flying by, and people were already thinking about autumn. My book was coming along nicely.

And then just as I was relaxing - icy cold water was thrown in my face.

In November, Andrew was told he needed tests because something had been flagged up on a check MRI scan.

I'm On My Way

Andrew was set to have a biopsy to confirm that what was shown on the scan was scarring and not cancer. There was no need to put him back on to chemo pills if he didn't have cancer. His body had been through enough, and the pills were completely unnecessary if all he had was scarring. He was booked in on the 23rd of November for a pre-consultation about the biopsy. He was staying strong and going through the motions, trying to be optimistic.

I went straight back to the studio to record the song 'Trust Me' For Andrew.

I told him I would sing a song every day to encourage him. I picked songs that meant something to us and songs that were encouraging.

On the 1st December, to be sure there were no cancer cells and that any other corporals on a scan were just scaring Andrew went to surgery. I had no idea if I would ever hear from him again. I had never spoken to his family before. I didn't know if I should contact them or just wait for Andrew to contact me.

We had always been in our own bubble, and neither of us really connected our families or anyone else in our lives together. We just had our own unique and special world, together.

While Andrew was in his operation, I was making plans to fly out to see him. I needed some help with the flight and hotel cost as I didn't have that kind of money. I asked people if they could help donate to a 'Fund Me' page. It took some swallowing of my pride, but it was worth it. I would only be going for a few days, but I desperately wanted to be there to see him.

On the 2nd of December, he texted me. I had never been so happy to see my phone flash. He said he was OK. It was tough for him to speak, and he was really weak, but he was OK.

The relief was tremendous. He said he would be in touch once he had some rest.

A few days later, Andrew called via WhatsApp. He said he was OK but still couldn't speak very loudly. It sounded like he had a hoarse voice and he had to strain to talk. He said he would have to wait at least a week before the results of the biopsy.

I told him I had started a 'Fund Me' page to get myself out there to see him. He was blown away, and I knew he was glad to hear it. I explained I just needed to raise funds for a flight and to get some money to stay at a hotel next door to the hospital.

While we were waiting for his results, we just carried on talking, and I tried so hard to be the same and not show my worry. His voice was getting weaker every day as it got harder for him to talk. I did all the talking and talked about all kinds of random things.

On the 12th December, I waited for the news of Andrews's appointment about the biopsy.

Being, the impatient person I was, I sent a message to just ask how he was getting on. He said 'OK'. I messaged him back to tell that I was so happy, and he wrote back with a smiley face.

I was elated again and couldn't wait to speak to him a bit more, later that day.

And to talk about my visit to see him.

Then a few hours later, Andrew texts to say he was sorry, he wasn't OK. The biopsy had shown he had cancer again. He said he hadn't known how to tell me earlier. The cancer was very aggressive, and there was nothing more to offer him in the way of treatment.

I felt faint and utterly gutted. I knew this was not the time to call him as he would be speaking to his family. I didn't want to cause any stress by trying to talk to him with questions about what the doctors would do now.

What I really wanted to ask was, 'How long do you have?'.

I reached out to his good friends who he had told me about many times in the past as he lived with them earlier that year. They were like family to him. I felt it would have been inappropriate to reach out to Andrew's brother or sisters, or mother. But I needed to speak to someone.

I reached out to his friends.

They were so helpful and thankfully they knew who I was. They were able to keep me up to date on his progress.

Everyone was desperately trying to get their head around the situation.
Before I knew it, it was Christmas. I was so grateful that Andrew was still able to understand and that although he was fatigued, his mind was still sharp.

My Brother and Phoebe flew in on the Christmas Eve to spend Christmas with us. It was a strange Christmas, typically one of my favourite times of the year. We did have some wonderful news that Phoebe was pregnant, and we would have a new Baby Bullimore arriving in the summer.

Andrew was sending me photos all the time and text messages that were a little jumbled up, but mostly I could understand them. We spent most of Christmas sending each other Emojis and pictures of whatever we were doing.

I had managed to raise £697 for my Flight and somewhere to stay in Rhode Island. I was looking for cheap flights and accommodation, and we planned for me to go out in early February.

I was so grateful to the people who were helping me to go and be with Andrew.

All I wanted to do was get there, but my body had different plans.

On the 23rd of January, I woke up feeling very odd. I needed to get up and go to my CBT therapist. I got on the bus, and some drunk man was shouting at the passengers that 'everyone was horrible'.

I usually wouldn't care about that, but he was unnerving me, and I was shaky and anxious and very faint.

I looked out the window and realised I'd gone past my bus stop and was at least 10 minutes down the road. I rang my mum to say I didn't feel right and tell her what had happened.

I said I would still try and get to my appointment. I hadn't seen my CBT man for over a month, and I really wanted to see him. I said I'd get there somehow.

I managed to get to an underground tube and make my way. I felt horrible. I wasn't sure if I should really just go home instead.

I got on the tube, and it was so hot and stuffy. Within 5 minutes of the journey, I thought, 'Crap I'm going to faint'.

There was a girl next to me, and I said very calmly.

"I know this is a little weird but, I am not feeling good. Could you help me if I faint?"

She was a lovely girl, and she gave me a can of Lemon fizz that I thought might help as it might be low blood sugar.

She helped me get off the tube at that point at what happened to be my stop. I said I was feeling better and the drink had helped. I said goodbye and called Mum again. I told her what had happened and that I was walking to the appointment at Kings Cross.

I made it to my appointment, and I told the CBT man I was not feeling at all well. I am pretty sure he probably thought it was just an anxiety attack.

After the appointment, I went to look for some food and more sugar. I was feeling so dizzy.

I managed to eat something and slowly make my way to the tube again. I got off at Brixton, and I suddenly had the terrifying feeling that I was going to have a seizure. I was petrified. I ended up getting an ambulance at Brixton, and I was rushed to the hospital.

I couldn't believe how weak I was and so dizzy and faint. I couldn't speak, and I was so scared.

Doctors said there was no apparent reason why it had happened but that it might be medication related and I should go to my specialist to discuss it as soon as I could.

I couldn't believe my health had let me down again. I was so anxious about being alone, in public. I was petrified to go out the house.
I very soon realised that there was no way I could get to Andrew. If I went, I would not be able to take care of myself, besides which, I was now frightened to go out in case I had another episode.

I kept Andrew completely up to date, and I had to tell him that I didn't know how I would get there or how I could cope alone. Andrew and I continued to talk and text.

I had raised the money, but now I sent an email to all the donors explaining what had happened. I said I would refund everyone's money to their accounts that day. With typical and utterly touching kindness they all said that I should give the money to Andrew for medical costs or any finance he may be struggling with.

On the 28th of January Andrew called me.

He said he was scared, and it broke my heart. I never once showed my concerns. I just tried to stay the same person I had always been. I didn't really know how else to behave. We talked, well, in reality, I spoke of how God was with him 100 percent, and he had nothing to fear. As Christians, we knew where we are going. We were praying and asking for strength.

When we got to the end of the conversation, I said, 'I love you', he said, 'I love you too' and told him that I would speak to him soon.

Now it seemed that I always had tears in my eyes and was just waiting for news.

Andrew rang again on the 29th, and I did some talking, but he said nothing. I know he rang, but I have no idea now if he understood anything, I said to him. When he hung up that day, I felt that it might be the last time I ever heard his breathing.

On the 7th of February, Andrew passed away. He was gone from his body, but I knew where his soul was. It was with God.

Aunty M Brain Tumours

I had never felt so broken. I had never lost a person so close to me that was so young. I had this aching empty gap in my life. It was numbing.

What did I do now, should I go to the States and go to the funeral? Then again, how could I? I was still so unwell, and I had given all the donated money to Andrews fundraiser.

Who could I talk to now that Andrew was gone? I never really discussed my friendship with Andrew with anyone else. They knew we were dating at one point, but I never shared that we still had a very close connection. I am a very private person and don't talk about my personal life regarding friends or family. It's just not something I do.

Maybe I should have spoken more about him to my friends? It was a week before Andrew's funeral was held. I felt absolutely lost.

The 14th of February was Andrew's Funeral. I did speak to one of Andrew's friends who texted me as he travelled to the funeral. He actually texted me through the service and told me what was being said. He took a picture of Andrew in the coffin. His friend was near the back of the church, so he wasn't close up, but I could see lots of people were there, and Andrew looked peaceful as though he was asleep in the open coffin.

I wasn't sure if it was right that Andrew's friend should be sending messages to me during the ceremony or a photo, but at the same time, it did help me to feel like I was there. I cried with everyone, and I said goodbye with everyone who loved Andrew.

After, the funeral, I was left with a feeling of 'Now what?'

I needed to grieve, and I needed to get my health right.

I had gone to see the Sleep Specialist again the following week to discuss my current symptoms. My mother came everywhere with me now as I was very disorientated and very unsteady on my legs. I was very weary and dizzy.

I asked if my current problems were medicine related? Were my symptoms normal?

She suggested I changed my medication and try something else. It would take some time to get it right, but I wasn't to worry about my symptoms, they would go once I was on the correct dosage.

Through all the waiting for appointments and for the medication to be sorted, I found it was vital to have a goal to distract me and to stop me focusing on the negative.

I started to get back onto my Aunty M Brain Tumours Website and decided to change it to a WordPress Blog. It was a way to carry on interviewing other people affected by brain tumours and encouraging others.

I have no idea what will happen to me in the future but what I do know is that I will always know I have been to hell and back and I can fight anything that is thrown at me.

Watch Out World!! Here I come!

Printed in Great Britain
by Amazon

48183524R00154